FOCUS ON
SLEEP MEDICINE

A SELF-ASSESSMENT

FOCUS ON SLEEP MEDICINE

A SELF-ASSESSMENT

Teofilo Lee-Chiong

W. David Brown

John Harrington

Max Hirshkowitz

James M. Parish

Leon Rosenthal

Francoise J. Roux

Daniel R. Smith

Sheila Tsai

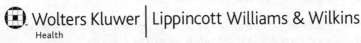
Wolters Kluwer | Lippincott Williams & Wilkins
Health

Philadelphia • Baltimore • New York • London
Buenos Aires • Hong Kong • Sydney • Tokyo

Acquisitions Editor: Lisa McAllister
Product Manager: Tom Gibbons
Manufacturing Manager: Ben Rivera
Marketing Manager: Brian Freiland
Cover Designer: Steve Druding
Production Service: Macmillan Publishing Solutions

Printed in China

Library of Congress Cataloging-in-Publication Data
Lee-Chiong, Teofilo, 1960-
    Focus on sleep medicine / Teofilo Lee-Chiong
        p. ; cm. —   (Neurology self-assessment)
    Includes index.
    ISBN-13: 978-1-58255-855-4
    ISBN-10: 1-58255-855-8
    1. Sleep disorders—Examinations, questions, etc. I. Title. II. Series: Neurology self-assessment.
    [DNLM: 1. Sleep Disorders—physiopathology—Examination Questions. 2. Neurology—
methods—Examination Questions. 3. Sleep Disorders—complications—Examination Questions.
Wl 18.2 L477f 2010]
    RC547.L437 2010
    616.8'4980076—dc22

                                                                2009015204

Care has been taken to confirm the accuracy of the information presented and to describe generally
accepted practices. However, the authors, editors, and publisher are not responsible for errors or
omissions or for any consequences from application of the information in this book and make no
warranty, expressed or implied, with respect to the currency, completeness, or accuracy of the
contents of the publication. Application of the information in a particular situation remains the
professional responsibility of the practitioner.

The authors, editors, and publisher have exerted every effort to ensure that drug selection and
dosage set forth in this text are in accordance with current recommendations and practice at the
time of publication. However, in view of ongoing research, changes in government regulations, and
the constant flow of information relating to drug therapy and drug reactions, the reader is urged to
check the package insert for each drug for any change in indications and dosage and for added
warnings and precautions. This is particularly important when the recommended agent is a new or
infrequently employed drug.

Some drugs and medical devices presented in the publication have Food and Drug
Administration (FDA) clearance for limited use in restricted research settings. It is the responsibility
of the health care provider to ascertain the FDA status of each drug or device planned for use in
their clinical practice.

To purchase additional copies of this book, call our customer service department at (800) 638-3030
or fax orders to (301) 223-2320. International customers should call (301) 223-2300.

Visit Lippincott Williams & Wilkins on the Internet: at LWW.com. Lippincott Williams & Wilkins
customer service representatives are available from 8:30 am to 6 pm, EST.

10 9 8 7 6 5 4 3 2 1

EDITORS

Teofilo Lee-Chiong, MD
Head, Division of Sleep Medicine
Department of Medicine
National Jewish Health
Denver, Colorado
Associate Professor of Medicine
University of Colorado Denver School of Medicine
Denver, Colorado

W. David Brown, PhD
Director
The Woodlands Sleep Evaluation Center
The Woodlands, Texas

John Harrington, MD, MPH
Assistant Professor of Medicine
Division of Sleep Medicine
National Jewish Health
Denver, Colorado

Max Hirshkowitz, PhD
Professor
Houston VA Medical Center
Houston, Texas

James M. Parish, MD
Associate Professor of Medicine
College of Medicine, Mayo Clinic
Chair, Division of Pulmonary Medicine
Department of Internal Medicine
Mayo Clinic Arizona
Scottsdale, Arizona

Leon Rosenthal, MD
Sleep Medicine Associates of Texas
Dallas, Texas

Francoise J. Roux, MD, PhD
Assistant Professor of Medicine
Department of Pulmonary and Critical Care Medicine
Yale University School of Medicine
Associate Director
Yale Center for Sleep Disorders
New Haven, Connecticut

Daniel R. Smith, MD
Assistant Professor of Medicine
Division of Sleep Medicine
Department of Medicine
National Jewish Health
Denver, Colorado

Sheila Tsai, MD
Assistant Professor of Medicine
Division of Sleep Medicine
Department of Medicine
National Jewish Health
Denver, Colorado

Sleep disorders, as an important clinical field, has slowly but steadily gained traction over the past 40 years. After decades of effort, sleep disorders medicine recently became a formally recognized medical specialty. The Accreditation Council for Graduate Medical Education (ACGME) now accredits sleep medicine fellowship training programs, and the American Board of Internal Medicine (ABIM) and American Board of Psychiatry and Neurology (ABPN) administer qualifying board examinations. These developments create the need for concise, focused, durable educational materials. Many "students" greatly value "instruction by example". When preparing for examination, what better example is there than sample questions? For this obvious reason, such books are quite popular in many fields. Consequently, this volume was conceived as a study aid for individuals interested in sharpening their didactic skills, especially in the process of preparing for the board examination.

Rather than rushing out a book of questions, we decided to wait until more specific information became available about the examination. The ABIM web site is very helpful in this regard. It breaks down the examination into specific topics and provides estimated constituent percentages. The examination has now been administered and one thing seems certain—the questions posed are not controversial. Each question is clearly evidence-based and derived from published clinical or scientific literature. Apparently some questions are straightforward but many are derivative, i.e., the answer relates to a presupposed conclusion drawn from the information provided. For example, a symptom constellation provided in a clinical case format clearly indicates that the patient has congestive heart failure (without ever mentioning the actual diagnosis). The question, however, relates to what type of breathing pattern might be revealed by polysomnography. Thus, one must recognize the underlying disorder in order to derive Cheyne-Stokes respiration as the associated sleep-disordered breathing pattern. In developing material for this volume, we attempted to format questions in both straightforward and derived configurations.

This book represents the efforts of experts from different areas of sleep medicine. Sleep medicine's multidisciplinary nature spans the spectrum of clinical specialties (Internal Medicine, Pulmonary Medicine, Neurology, Psychiatry, Pediatrics, Surgery, Dentistry, and Psychology). It also cuts across, and includes, more global categories such as aging, gender, neurophysiology, pharmacology, dreaming, sleep deprivation, and standards of practice. Finally, several questions address methodology, instrumentation, and technique. We, the authors, have tried our best to represent all of these topics.

Our process was simple. First, we listed relevant topics indicated on the board examination sites and that the group deemed important. Next, we developed questions related to each topic and assigned each to an author. That author refined the question's wording, created an answer set, designated a correct answer, and wrote an explanation indicating why that answer was correct (and why the others were wrong). These items were then reviewed by one or more of the other editors. Finally, the entirety of material was organized and now sits before you. We hope you find this useful for your study and review. And most of all . . . good luck.

Teofilo Lee-Chiong
W. David Brown
John Harrington
Max Hirshkowitz
James M. Parish
Leon Rosenthal
Francoise J. Roux
Daniel R. Smith
Sheila Tsai

CONTENTS

SECTION 1

Questions

1. **Which of the following statements regarding sleep in the elderly compared to younger persons is most correct?**
   A. Older adults have shortened latency to sleep onset, decreased wake time after sleep onset (WASO), and increased N3 sleep
   B. Older adults have prolonged latency to sleep onset, increased WASO, and reduced N3 sleep
   C. Older adults have shortened sleep latency to sleep onset, decreased WASO, and increased N3 sleep
   D. Older adults have prolonged latency to sleep onset, increased WASO, and increased N3 sleep

2. **A 42-year-old woman reports brief terrifying episodes of being unable to move when she awakens from sleep. She denies symptoms of daytime sleepiness. Which of the following statements regarding sleep paralysis is correct?**
   A. This phenomenon occurs in approximately 90% of narcoleptic patients
   B. Visual, but not auditory or tactile, hallucinations may occur during episodes
   C. Episodes of sleep paralysis typically last for 1 hour
   D. It is a component of the classic tetrad of narcolepsy, which includes excessive daytime sleepiness, cataplexy, and hypnagogic hallucinations

3. **The stimulant effects of caffeine are primarily mediated through antagonism of which central nervous system (CNS) receptor?**
   A. Gamma aminobutyric acid (GABA)
   B. Norepinephrine
   C. Adenosine
   D. Dopamine

4. **Which of the following medications is associated with the artifact noted in Figure 1?**
   A. Bupropion
   B. Zolpidem
   C. Modafinil
   D. Fluoxetine

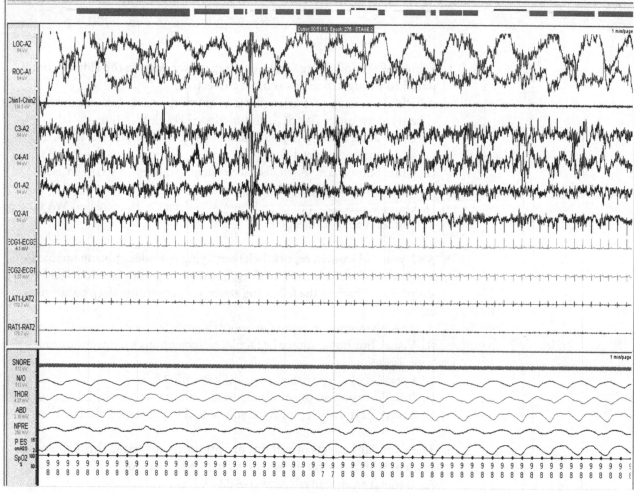

Figure 1.

5. **Which of the following features is associated with sleep-related groaning or catathrenia?**
   A. Epileptiform discharges on electroencephalography
   B. Night-to-night consistency in presentation and severity
   C. Significant sleep disturbance with frequent awakenings
   D. Inspiratory moaning or groaning

6. **Which of the following represents the location and observed findings of Frédérick Bremer's cerveau isolé preparation?**
   A. Transection in the lower medulla resulting in electroencephalographic manifestations of persistent wakefulness
   B. Transection at the level of the midbrain immediately caudal to the oculomotor nerves, resulting in electroencephalographic features consistent with persistent sleep
   C. Transection in the lower medulla resulting in electroencephalographic features consistent with persistent sleep
   D. Transection at the level of the midbrain immediately caudal to the oculomotor nerves, resulting in electroencephalographic manifestations of alternating sleep and wakefulness

7. **Positron emission tomography (PET) imaging studies involving patients with insomnia have suggested which of the following features?**
   A. Decreased cerebral metabolism in wake-promoting regions from waking to sleep states
   B. Increased cerebral metabolism during NREM sleep
   C. Increased prefrontal cortex metabolism during wakefulness
   D. Increased wake time after sleep onset (WASO) related to decreased thalamocortical and pontine metabolism

8. **A patient has severe restless legs syndrome. She has recently increased her daily dose of levodopa/carbidopa to 200/50 mg at bedtime because of worsening symptoms. She now reports that she is experiencing symptoms much earlier in the day and that her latency to symptom onset has shortened. Which of the following terms correctly identifies this phenomenon?**
   A. Tolerance
   B. Rebound
   C. Dependency
   D. Augmentation

9. **Which of the following antidepressants is most likely to suppress REM sleep?**
   A. Paroxetine
   B. Trazodone
   C. Doxepin
   D. Phenelzine

10. **A 36-year-old man with bipolar disorder is referred to the sleep laboratory for symptoms of excessive daytime somnolence. An overnight polysomnogram fails to demonstrate a primary sleep disorder and his symptoms are attributed to lithium carbonate use. Which of the following is commonly associated with this medication?**
    A. Decreased total sleep time
    B. Decreased REM sleep
    C. Decreased stage N3 sleep
    D. Insomnia and significant reduction in sleep efficiency

11. **A 43-year-old man with severe obstructive sleep apnea presents to the sleep clinic with complaints of persistent hypersomnolence. He states that he uses continuous positive airway pressure (CPAP) every night for at least 6 hours per night. The compliance download from his device corroborates his report. A CPAP titration performed at his prescribed pressure reduces the apnea–hypopnea index (AHI) to 3.0 per hour and maintained oxygen saturation above 90%. No other causes of sleepiness are identified. Which of the following statements is correct regarding adjunctive modafinil therapy?**
    A. It does not affect CPAP compliance
    B. Common side effects include headache and nausea
    C. Dependence and tolerance are frequently observed
    D. It adversely affects nighttime sleep quality after morning intake

12. A 17-year-old male presents to the sleep clinic for evaluation of episodes of excessive sleepiness. The patient's mother reports that he has had several episodes of prolonged sleep time intermittently over the last year. Which of the following is associated with Kleine–Levin syndrome?
    A. Sleepiness tends to diminish in severity over time
    B. Decreased food intake and weight loss
    C. Persistent excessive sleepiness
    D. Cataplexy-like symptoms

13. A 36-year-old woman reports almost nightly episodes of excessive food intake. She often has no recall of the event the following morning but may find crumbs or food wrappers in her bed. She has complained of recent weight gain. Her husband reports that she eats whatever she can find and has even consumed frozen foods or inedible items on occasion. Which primary sleep disorder is most commonly associated with this condition?
    A. Night terrors
    B. Rhythmic movement disorder
    C. Sleepwalking
    D. Narcolepsy

14. A 19-year-old college freshman presents to the sleep clinic during her summer break. She complains that during the previous academic year, she had great difficulty falling asleep before 2:00 a.m. or arising on time for her morning classes. After further assessment and reviewing her sleep diary, you diagnose her as having delayed sleep phase syndrome (DSPS). Since she has several weeks before the next term begins, she is interested in a trial of chronotherapy. Which of the following statements regarding chronotherapy is correct?
    A. Attempts to resynchronize the individual's circadian rhythm with the 24-hour light–dark cycle
    B. Always utilizes progressive delay of the sleep–wake schedule
    C. Results are predictable, long-lasting, and resistant
    D. More effective for advanced sleep phase syndrome

15. Which of the following statements regarding sleep associated with alcohol abstinence is most accurate?
    A. Sleep disturbances may persist even after prolonged abstinence
    B. Decreased REM density at 6 months highly correlates with relapse
    C. Baseline sleep efficiency is a predictor of alcohol relapse after treatment
    D. Polysomnographic features noted early following abstinence include prolonged sleep latencies, reduced total sleep time, and decreased REM sleep

16. A 37-year-old gentleman presents to his primary care physician with complaints of insomnia for several months. On further questioning, the patient admits to staying up late frequently because he is either surfing the Internet or playing computer games. During these periods, he drinks caffeinated sodas. If he goes to bed earlier, he typically watches television for several hours before falling asleep. He reports that his sleep–wake

schedule is quite variable and that he may stay awake until as late as 3 a.m. a few days each week. He always gets out of bed by 8 a.m. to go to work, but because of sleepiness, he often takes long naps in the late afternoon or early evening after work and commonly sleeps into the early afternoon on weekends. On evenings after long naps, he describes difficulty falling asleep. He states that when he occasionally refrains from watching television or using his computer, he falls asleep typically by 11 p.m. and awakens at 7:30 a.m. spontaneously. His symptoms are not generally affected by travel. He denies symptoms suggestive of obstructive sleep apnea, restless legs syndrome, or mood disorder. This patient's history is most consistent with which of the following disorders?

A. Delayed sleep phase syndrome
B. Psychophysiologic insomnia
C. Environmental sleep disorder
D. Inadequate sleep hygiene

17. **Which of the following regarding nonentrained circadian rhythm disorder is correct?**

A. This disorder is more common among blind persons
B. There is a progressive advance in sleep–wake periods over time
C. Manifested sleep–wake cycle is typically slightly shorter than 24 hours
D. Bright light exposure is usually the first-line therapy for this disorder

18. **Which sleep disorder is characterized by variable sleep periods that lack an identifiable circadian rhythm?**

A. Irregular sleep–wake rhythm
B. Delayed sleep phase syndrome
C. Free-running sleep disorder
D. Recurrent hypersomnia

19. **Obstructive sleep apnea is prevalent among children with Down syndrome. Which of the following anatomic abnormalities is typically identified as a risk factor in these patients?**

A. Midfacial hypoplasia
B. Microglossia
C. Widened palate
D. Macrognathia

20. **Which of the following statements regarding sleep in blind persons is true?**

A. Blind persons report more sleep complaints compared to sighted persons
B. Free-running circadian disorder is the most common sleep disorder among blind persons
C. Persons without light perception invariably display circadian desynchrony
D. Melatonin is not an effective entrainment therapy for circadian rhythm abnormalities in blind persons

21. **What is the cardiac rhythm represented in the following figure?**
    A. Sinus bradycardia
    B. First-degree atrioventricular (AV) block
    C. Ventricular escape
    D. Paced rhythm

A
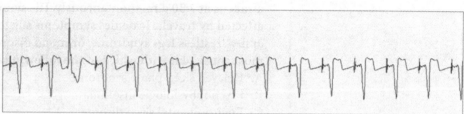

B
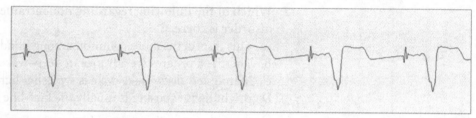

Figure 2.

22. **Histaminergic nuclei are located primarily in which area of the brain?**
    A. Locus coeruleus
    B. Perifornical neurons of the lateral hypothalamus
    C. Basal forebrain
    D. Tuberomammillary nucleus of the posterior hypothalamus

23. **A 23-year-old woman is undergoing a multiple sleep latency test for evaluation of her complaints of severe daytime sleepiness. The second nap period began ("lights out") at 10:05 a.m. Sleep onset was recorded at 10:15 a.m. The following sleep epoch (see Fig. 3) is recorded at 10:18 a.m. Which of the following statements regarding this nap opportunity is correct?**
    A. REM sleep latency is 3 minutes
    B. The nap period should end at 10:32 a.m.
    C. REM sleep latency is 13 minutes
    D. The nap period should end at 10:25 a.m.

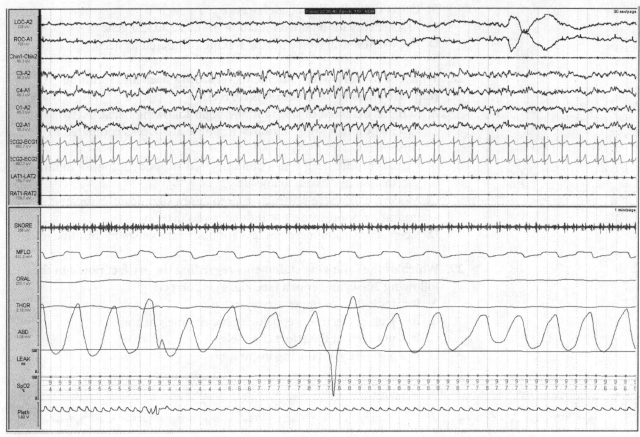

Figure 3.

24. **Which of the following features is associated with fatal familial insomnia?**
    A. Anterior ventral and dorsomedial thalamic nuclei degeneration
    B. Hereditary form due to a single point mutation at codon 180 of the *PRNP* gene
    C. Female preponderance
    D. Autosomal recessive mode of transmission

25. **Which neural structure is the primary generator of sleep spindles?**
    A. Suprachiasmatic nucleus
    B. Lateral hypothalamus
    C. Thalamic reticular nucleus
    D. Locus coeruleus

26. **Gastric acid secretion demonstrates a circadian rhythmicity. When does peak gastric acid secretion occur?**
    A. 6 p.m. to 10 p.m.
    B. 10 a.m. to 2 p.m.
    C. 6 a.m. to 10 p.m.
    D. 10 p.m. to 2 a.m.

27. **Which of the following statements regarding congenital central alveolar hypoventilation syndrome (CCHS) is correct?**
    A. Mechanical ventilation during wakefulness is generally required even in mild disease

B. Onset typically during adolescence

C. Associated with de novo mutation in the *PHOX2B* gene

D. Hypoventilation worse during waking compared to sleep

28. **Which of the following statements regarding sleep and immune responsiveness to vaccination is correct?**
    A. Subjects deprived of sleep for one night following hepatitis A vaccination had lower antibody response at 4 weeks compared to controls
    B. Partial chronic sleep restriction impaired antibody response to influenza vaccination at 3-week follow-up
    C. Moderate to severe obstructive sleep apnea significantly impairs immune responsiveness to influenza vaccination
    D. Sleep deprivation increases IgG antibody catabolism in immune mice

29. **Which of the following statements regarding the artifact noted in the following 30-second epoch (see Fig. 4) is correct?**
    A. It is indicative of upper airway patency
    B. It is seen in electroencephalographic channels as well
    C. It is not seen in the effort channels
    D. It is also observed during inspiration

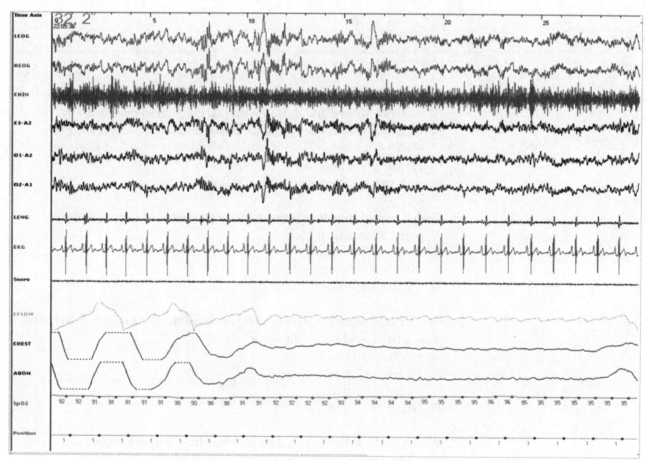

Figure 4.

30. **Which of the following statements best describes restless legs syndrome?**
    A. Numbness and tingling sensation in the lower extremities
    B. Sensation of inner restlessness with a desire to move the entire body
    C. Continuous undulating movement of the toes
    D. Disagreeable sensation in the legs that is worse in the evening and at rest, and relieved by activity

31. **Which of these conditions is associated with restless legs syndrome?**
    A. Thalassemia
    B. Iron deficiency anemia
    C. Polymyalgia rheumatica
    D. Fibromyalgia

32. **Which of the following medications has been implicated in worsening restless legs syndrome symptoms?**
    A. Benzodiazepines
    B. Opioid narcotics
    C. Selective serotonin reuptake inhibitors
    D. Bupropion

33. **Which of the following best describes the effect of alcohol on sleep?**
    A. Delays sleep latency
    B. Shortens sleep latency
    C. Increases REM sleep
    D. Decreases NREM sleep

34. **Which of the following statements regarding sleep during pregnancy is correct?**
    A. Incidence of snoring is increased
    B. Incidence of sleep-disordered breathing is decreased
    C. Elevated estrogen levels decrease the risk of upper airway resistance syndrome
    D. Elevated levels of progesterone cause upper airway edema

35. **What is the effect of acute cocaine administration on sleep?**
    A. REM latency is decreased
    B. Sleep latency is increased
    C. Delta sleep is decreased
    D. Percentage of REM sleep is decreased

36. **Which of the following medications bind to the alpha-1 subunit of the gamma aminobutyric acid (GABA)-A receptor complex?**
    A. Ramelteon
    B. Quazepam
    C. Zaleplon
    D. Trazodone

37. **Which of the following medications is alerting and can cause insomnia?**
    A. Gamma hydroxybutyrate
    B. Theophylline
    C. Lamotrigine
    D. Amitriptyline

38. **Which of the following medications is associated with excessive daytime somnolence?**
    A. Modafinil
    B. Bupropion
    C. Captopril
    D. Amitriptyline

39. **Which of the following neurologic conditions is most closely associated with REM sleep behavior disorder?**
    A. Parkinson disease
    B. Alzheimer disease
    C. Seizure disorder
    D. Post-polio syndrome

40. **Acute sleep deprivation can lead to which of the following?**
    A. Increased leptin level
    B. Increased ghrelin level
    C. Decreased cortisol level
    D. Decreased thyroid-stimulating hormone (TSH) concentrations

41. **Compared to tonic REM sleep, phasic REM sleep is associated with which of the following?**
    A. Decreased sympathetic activity
    B. Increased sympathetic activity
    C. Decreased parasympathetic activity
    D. Increased sympathetic and parasympathetic activity

42. **60-Hz artifact is due to which of the following?**
    A. Faulty electrode placement
    B. Excessive sweating
    C. Movement of the patient
    D. Electrode impedance lower than 1,000 Ω

43. **A 65-year-old male was diagnosed with severe obstructive sleep apnea. He was started on continuous positive airway pressure (CPAP) at 10 cm H_2O 1 month ago. He reports that he is feeling better but is still sleepy at times. He complains of a dry mouth sensation in the morning and finds the CPAP mask off upon awakening in the morning. He has no symptoms of restless legs and his polysomnography does not show any increase in periodic leg movements during sleep. What is the best intervention at this time?**
    A. Serial contacts by phone
    B. Increase total sleep time
    C. Mask-fitting session
    D. Application of nasal saline spray before bedtime

44. A 55-year-old man has severe obstructive sleep apnea (OSA) with an apnea–hypopnea index (AHI) of 55 and oxygen desaturation as low as 72%. He refuses treatment for his OSA. He is at increased risk for which of the following?
    A. Stroke
    B. Ventricular tachycardia
    C. Sudden cardiac death
    D. Hypercapnia

45. Alpha electroencephalographic wave intrusions are usually seen during which of the following?
    A. REM sleep only
    B. NREM sleep
    C. N3 sleep only
    D. N2 sleep only

46. A 35-year-old male is treated for anxiety and depression. His electroencephalographic tracing during polysomnography reveals frequent pseudo-spindles. Which of the following medications is he taking?
    A. Selective serotonin reuptake inhibitor
    B. Neuroleptic agent
    C. Atypical antidepressant
    D. Benzodiazepine

47. A 22-year-old man is complaining of excessive daytime somnolence since he started a new job several months ago. He goes to bed at 2:00 a.m. and has to get up early in the morning for work. His score on the Epworth Sleepiness Scale is 13/24 indicative of significant hypersomnia. He denies any symptoms of cataplexy but reports occasional sleep paralysis. Polysomnography does not reveal any sleep-disordered breathing or movement disorder. Multiple sleep latency tests shows a mean sleep latency of 10 minutes with two sleep-onset REM periods. What is the most likely cause of his excessive daytime somnolence?
    A. Narcolepsy without cataplexy
    B. Idiopathic hypersomnia
    C. Delayed sleep phase syndrome
    D. Depression

48. Compared to healthy individuals, heart rate variability in patients with severe obstructive sleep apnea is characterized by which of the following?
    A. Heart rate variability is related to decreased sympathetic nervous system activity during an apneic episode
    B. Increased heart rate variability is associated with adverse cardiovascular events
    C. Decreased heart rate variability is associated with adverse cardiovascular events
    D. Heart rate variability is inversely correlated to disease severity

49. **Which of the following antidepressants is the most sedating?**
    A. Fluoxetine
    B. Paroxetine
    C. Fluvoxamine
    D. Sertraline

50. **A 35-year-old woman has been taking triazolam at bedtime for insomnia for the last 3 months. Her primary care physician discontinues the triazolam and switches her to ramelteon believing that ramelteon has fewer side effects. She now complains of worsening insomnia. She is most likely suffering from which of the following?**
    A. Acute anxiety
    B. Side effects from ramelteon
    C. Benzodiazepine withdrawal
    D. Rebound insomnia

51. **A 19-year-old male reports jaw discomfort in the morning. His wife describes an unpleasant noise when he clenches and grinds his teeth at night. Which of the following statements regarding bruxism is correct?**
    A. Relieved by muscle relaxants and alcohol
    B. Severity diminished by selective serotonin reuptake inhibitor (SSRI)
    C. Most frequent during stage N3 sleep
    D. Can present as sudden increase in electroencephalographic activity

52. **A 62-year-old man comes to the sleep clinic at the request of his wife. She reports that he recently started kicking and punching her in his sleep. She is adamant that there is no marital discord but is scared of his violent behavior. When she wakes him up, he can recall a terrible dream where he was in a fight and had to defend himself. What is the most likely diagnosis?**
    A. Sleep terrors
    B. Posttraumatic stress disorder
    C. REM sleep behavior disorder
    D. Seizure disorder

53. **Body rocking is a parasomnia that is associated with which of the following?**
    A. Occurs only in children
    B. Occurs during drowsiness and resolves during sleep
    C. Is more common in children with mental retardation
    D. Commonly requires treatment with benzodiazepines to prevent injury

54. **Sleepwalking generally occurs during which of the following?**
    A. The last third of the night
    B. The first third of the night
    C. REM sleep
    D. Drowsiness and stage N1 sleep

55. **Which of the following statements regarding periodic leg movements during sleep is correct?**
    A. Patients generally present with complaints of repetitive leg movements during sleep
    B. A periodic limb movement index greater than 15 should always be treated
    C. Prevalence is increased in patients with REM sleep behavior disorder
    D. They commonly respond to dopamine antagonists

56. **Which of the following statements best describes traumatic brain injury?**
    A. New onset of excessive daytime somnolence is more common than complaints of insomnia
    B. Objective measure of sleepiness (e.g., multiple sleep latency test) is generally normal
    C. New onset of sleep–wake disturbances is uncommon, affecting about 10% of patients with traumatic brain injury
    D. Cerebrospinal fluid levels of hypocretin are normal

57. **Which of the following statements concerning complex sleep apnea is true?**
    A. Development of central apneas during acute application of continuous positive airway pressure (CPAP) in obstructive sleep apnea patients with initially predominant obstructive apneic or hypopneic events
    B. Induced by cerebrovascular accidents
    C. A form of Cheyne–Stokes breathing
    D. Best treated with higher levels of CPAP

58. **Sleep deprivation has been associated with which of the following changes?**
    A. Increase in cellular immunity
    B. Increase in IL-1 level
    C. Decrease in interferon-alpha level
    D. Increase in IL-2 level

59. **Acute partial sleep deprivation is associated with which of the following changes in sleep architecture?**
    A. Increase in REM sleep
    B. Decrease in REM sleep
    C. Prolongation of sleep latency
    D. Decrease in stage N3 sleep

60. **Sleep deprivation is associated with which of the following?**
    A. Decreased level of ghrelin
    B. Impaired glucose tolerance test
    C. Decreased level of cortisol
    D. Elevated level of leptin

61. **Compared to levels during wakefulness, cerebral blood flow during sleep is best described by which of the following?**
    A. Increased during NREM sleep
    B. Unchanged during NREM sleep
    C. Increased during REM sleep
    D. Decreased during REM sleep

62. **An 85-year-old male complains that for the last couple of years, he feels sleepy and needs to go to bed around 8:00 p.m. His sleep latency is within 15 minutes. He denies any snoring or witnessed apneas. He wakes up once during the night to go to the bathroom but goes back to sleep quickly. His final rising time is 4:30 a.m. to 5:00 a.m. He is worried that he might not be getting enough sleep. He feels refreshed when he wakes up and starts gardening until he has breakfast with his wife at 9:00 a.m. He takes a nap at 1:00 p.m. for about 1 hour. He denies any symptoms of depression. He reports that his wife is very concerned when he wakes her up everyday at 5:00 a.m. and would like him to sleep longer. Which treatment would be the best for this patient?**
    A. Exposure to bright light in the morning
    B. Exposure to bright light in the evening
    C. Melatonin therapy in the evening
    D. Exposure to dim light in the evening

63. **Which of the following statements regarding myotonic dystrophy is true?**
    A. A distal myopathy that affects the pharyngeal and laryngeal musculature but spares the diaphragm
    B. Increased likelihood of central but not obstructive sleep apnea
    C. Increased risk of pulmonary hypertension
    D. Alveolar hypoventilation is worse during NREM sleep compared to REM sleep

64. **A 19-year-old man complains of sudden and brief contractions of one of his legs when he is trying to fall asleep. He has been studying for an examination and reports decreased total sleep time over the past 2 weeks compared to his usual schedule. He denies any unpleasant sensation or pain in his legs. He feels otherwise normal and has no other complaints. What is the likely diagnosis?**
    A. Periodic leg movement disorder
    B. Restless legs syndrome
    C. Muscle cramps
    D. Hypnic jerks

65. **Cognitive effects of sleep deprivation include which of the following?**
    A. Periods of hyperresponsiveness
    B. Decreased performance with increased time-on-task
    C. Increased cognitive performance
    D. Generalized increased rate of behavioral responses

66. A mildly obese 50-year-old man without known cardiac disease is referred for a diagnostic polysomnogram for symptoms of snoring and daytime fatigue. During the study, he demonstrates a pattern of mild apnea without significant oxygen desaturation. His electrocardiogram reveals normal sinus rhythm with variable heart rate changes and periods of bradycardia with 4-second sinus pauses during REM sleep. What is the appropriate response to this finding?
    A. Initiate cardiopulmonary resuscitation protocol for bradycardia
    B. Transport the patient to an emergency room by ambulance for evaluation
    C. Emergently notify the medical director of the sleep laboratory
    D. Continue with the testing

67. A 35-year-old-woman with complaints of insomnia presents for follow-up. She is noncompliant with maintaining a sleep log and continues to complain of poor sleep. A recent polysomnogram reveals markedly reduced sleep efficiency without evidence of sleep-disordered breathing or periodic limb activity. Which of the following may yield significant clinical data to assist in her management?
    A. A repeat polysomnogram
    B. Repeat polysomnography with multiple sleep latency test
    C. Maintenance of wakefulness testing
    D. Actigraphy

68. A 35-year-old overweight man presents for evaluation of snoring. His wife reports an increased frequency of snoring with no observed apneic events. His primary care physician recently performed an in-home overnight oximetry that reportedly revealed no evidence of significant oxygen desaturation. His physical examination is noteworthy for mildly redundant pharyngeal tissues and a blood pressure of 145/90. What is the best course of action?
    A. Perform a polysomnography
    B. Reassure the patient that no further evaluation is required
    C. Refer the patient to an otolaryngologist for uvulopalatopharyngoplasty
    D. Advise weight loss

69. Which of the following statements is true regarding use of the Epworth Sleepiness Scale (EES)?
    A. ESS scoring may be used to definitively diagnose narcolepsy
    B. ESS scores correlate well with multiple sleep latency test data
    C. A score of 10 or lower suggests pathologic daytime somnolence
    D. 25% of the general population may have a score of >12

70. What is the stage illustrated in Figure 5?
    A. REM sleep
    B. Stage W (Wake) with eyes opened
    C. Stage W (Wake) with eyes closed
    D. Stage 1 (N1) sleep

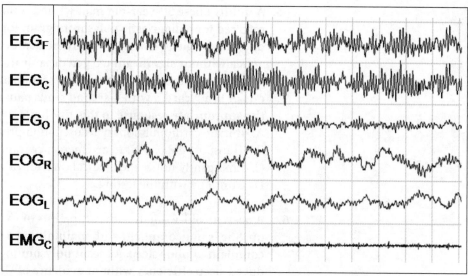

Figure 5.

71. **Which of the following statements is true regarding sleep bruxism?**
    A. It is most likely to occur during REM sleep
    B. It is associated with stress
    C. It does not cause significant dental pathology
    D. Therapy with selective serotonin reuptake inhibitors (SSRIs) is effective

72. **Which of the following contributes to the pathophysiology of central sleep apnea/Cheyne–Stokes respiration in congestive heart failure?**
    A. Increased use of beta-blockers
    B. Increased circulatory time
    C. Decreased respiratory drive
    D. Increased loop gain

73. **Which of the following statements about "overlap syndrome" is true?**
    A. It is a rare clinical condition
    B. Nocturnal oxygen alone is the best therapy
    C. It is usually seen in the setting of severe obstructive lung disease
    D. It is defined by the combination of obstructive sleep apnea and intrinsic lung disease

74. **Which of the following statements regarding upper airway resistance syndrome is correct?**
    A. Polysomnography data demonstrate an elevated apnea–hypopnea index (AHI)
    B. Nasal thermistors are required to detect subtle respiratory events
    C. Patients exhibit symptoms of daytime somnolence or fatigue
    D. Patients demonstrate significant episodic oxygen desaturations

75. **A normal weight man with mild obstructive sleep apnea, apnea–hypopnea index (AHI) of 12, and continuous positive airway pressure (CPAP) intolerance requests advice for alternative treatments for apnea. Which of the following would you recommend for this patient?**

A. Nocturnal nasal oxygen therapy
B. Uvulopalatopharyngoplasty (UPPP)
C. Mandibular advancement/oral appliance
D. Reassurance that no treatment is necessary for mild obstructive sleep apnea

76. **Which of the following is a recommendation for perioperative management of patients with obstructive sleep apnea?**
A. Postoperative screening to identify patients at risk for sleep apnea
B. Use of general anesthesia, if possible, instead of regional or spinal/epidural anesthesia
C. Use of supine positioning of patients
D. Continuous monitoring of respiratory parameters until full recovery from sedation

77. **What sleep stage is represented in the following epoch (see Fig. 6)?**
A. N1 sleep
B. N2 sleep
C. N3 sleep
D. REM sleep

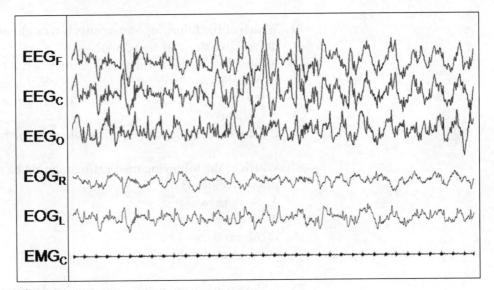

Figure 6.

78. **A 45-year-old man presents following a recent polysomnogram. He is mildly obese with borderline hypertension, daytime fatigue, and an Epworth Sleepiness Score of 12. His polysomnogram reveals an apnea–hypopnea index (AHI) of 6 without significant positional changes in the frequency of respiratory events. REM sleep is associated with an AHI of 30 with oxygen desaturations to 85%. An appropriate therapeutic intervention includes which of the following?**
A. Reassurance that a normal AHI warrants no treatment
B. Advice on weight loss and positional modification
C. Initiation of nocturnal oxygen at 2 L/min
D. Continuous positive airway pressure (CPAP) titration study

79. **Which of the following anatomical findings is associated with an increased risk of obstructive sleep apnea?**
    A. Macrognathia
    B. Elongated mandible
    C. Increased tongue tissue
    D. Anteriorly displaced hyoid bone

80. **A 38-year-old asymptomatic man presents for polysomnography (PSG) at his wife's insistence for snoring that disrupts her sleep. He is mildly overweight, normotensive, and denies symptoms of fatigue, poor sleep, or behavioral changes. His PSG reveals an apnea–hypopnea index of 9 and included supine REM sleep. Which of the following measures is most appropriate at this time?**
    A. Schedule a continuous positive airway pressure (CPAP) titration study immediately
    B. Refer to an otolaryngologist for surgical evaluation
    C. Recommend weight loss and behavioral changes and consider pursuing follow-up PSG to reassess on the basis of observed symptoms
    D. Reassure patient that his obstructive apnea is mild and needs no additional evaluation

81. **Which of the following statements is true about weight loss for obstructive sleep apnea (OSA)?**
    A. Weight loss alone will reliably eliminate mild OSA in all patients
    B. Weight loss is only effective for OSA in the morbidly obese population
    C. Modest weight loss may eliminate or lessen severity of OSA in some patients
    D. There is no role for weight loss alone in the management of OSA

82. **Which of the following medications should be used clinically to increase slow-wave sleep?**
    A. Sodium oxybate
    B. Olanzapine
    C. Alprazolam
    D. None of the above

83. **A 55-year-old woman with obstructive sleep apnea (OSA) returns for follow-up. She was diagnosed with OSA 2 years previously and underwent successful continuous positive airway pressure (CPAP) titration with effective pressures obtained for supine REM sleep. She initially experienced subjective improvements in daytime fatigue and somnolence, but now reports worsening symptoms despite continued CPAP compliance. Which of the following may explain her current symptoms?**
    A. Reduced CPAP compliance
    B. Weight gain
    C. Depression
    D. All of the above

84. **Patients with obstructive sleep apnea, as compared to people without apnea, have which pattern of upper airway motor activity in the awake state?**
    A. Increased tonic and phasic activity
    B. Decreased tonic and increased phasic activity
    C. Increased tonic and decreased phasic activity
    D. Decreased tonic and phasic activity

85. **A 25-year-old man with complaints of daytime fatigue undergoes a diagnostic polysomnogram. The study reveals primarily central apneas with mild associated oxygen desaturations. Which of the following medications might explain this finding?**
    A. Acetazolamide
    B. Methadone
    C. Alprazolam
    D. Digoxin

86. **Which of the following is associated with an increased risk for sudden infant death syndrome (SIDS)?**
    A. Low bedroom temperature
    B. Maternal smoking
    C. Female gender
    D. Supine sleep position

87. **A 4-year-old girl displays increased repetitive leg activity nightly that appears to be associated with some apparent discomfort. It also occasionally occurs at naptime and at other times of reduced activity. She does not reliably report any specific leg discomfort but appears to have less limb activity after moving or stretching. What is the most likely diagnosis?**
    A. Restless legs syndrome
    B. Frontal lobe seizures
    C. Fragmentary myoclonus
    D. Sleep starts or hypnic jerk

88. **Which of the following is the likely diagnosis for a 30-month-old child with problems going to bed and frequent nocturnal awakenings, and difficulty returning to sleep and problems going to bed without a parent remaining in the room?**
    A. Limit-setting sleep disorder
    B. Sleep-onset association disorder
    C. Restless legs syndrome
    D. Sleep enuresis

89. **A 27-year-old woman undergoing polysomnography awakens during REM sleep complaining of a pulsing unilateral headache and nausea. She reports to the night technician that she has had similar headaches that are worsened by bright lights. Which is the most likely cause of her symptoms?**
    A. Hypnic headache
    B. Cluster headache
    C. Migraine headache
    D. Exploding head syndrome

90. A 28-year-old man with chronic T6 paraplegia complains of poor sleep and morning headaches. A diagnostic polysomnogram reveals the presence of sleep-disordered breathing with an apnea–hypopnea index (AHI) of 17. What is the most appropriate intervention at this time?
    A. Reassure the patient that these findings are normal in spinal cord injury
    B. Initiate nocturnal oxygen to prevent oxygen desaturations during sleep
    C. Full-night continuous positive airway pressure (CPAP) titration study
    D. Perform tracheotomy and initiate full nocturnal ventilation

91. Which of the following cardiovascular changes occurs during NREM sleep compared to wakefulness?
    A. Decrease in heart rate
    B. Increase in renal circulation
    C. Decrease in coronary circulation
    D. No change in cardiac output

92. Which of the following neurotransmitters is associated mainly with the generation and maintenance of REM sleep?
    A. Hypocretin
    B. Acetylcholine
    C. Histamine
    D. Norepinephrine

93. Nocturnal secretion of which of the following hormones is influenced primarily by the circadian rhythm rather than by sleep itself?
    A. Thyroid-stimulating hormone
    B. Cortisol
    C. Growth hormone
    D. Prolactin

94. Which of the following cytokines has been shown to enhance sleep?
    A. Interleukin 1β
    B. Interleukin 4
    C. Interleukin 10
    D. Interleukin 13

95. Where are the neurons associated with the neurotransmitter dopamine primarily located?
    A. Substantia nigra
    B. Tuberomammillary nucleus of the posterior hypothalamus
    C. Locus coeruleus
    D. Ventrolateral preoptic area

96. Which of the following statements about sleep-related changes in thermoregulation is correct?
    A. Among healthy adults, minimum core body temperature occurs about 2 hours after the habitual wake time among healthy adults
    B. Sweating and shivering are absent during both NREM and REM sleep

C. Activity of warmth-sensing neurons increases at sleep onset

D. Initiating sleep during the falling phase of the temperature rhythm leads to an increase in sleep latency and decrease in total sleep time

97. **What sleep stage does the following 30-second epoch (see Fig. 7) represent?**
    A. Stage N1
    B. Stage N2
    C. Stage N3
    D. Stage R

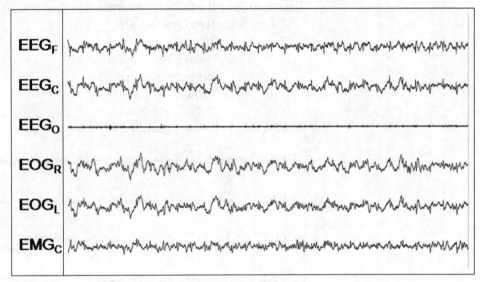

Figure 7.

98. **On the basis of the *2007 American Academy of Sleep Medicine Manual for the Scoring of Sleep and Associated Events,* which of the following is the recommended sensor for detecting apneas among adults?**
    A. Nasal pressure transducer
    B. Respiratory inductance plethysmography
    C. Esophageal manometry
    D. Oronasal thermal sensor

99. **Which of the following countermeasures is effective in enhancing alertness during night shift work in persons with shift work sleep disorder?**
    A. Administration of melatonin before daytime sleep following night shift work
    B. Scheduling phase advances (night to evening to day) rather than phase delays (night to day to evening) in shifts
    C. Use of hypnotic medications to shorten sleep latency and improve sleep efficiency during daytime sleep
    D. Exposure to bright lights in the workplace

100. **Which of the following statements regarding the maintenance of wakefulness test is correct?**
    A. An overnight polysomnography should always be performed on the evening immediately prior to the test
    B. A test is terminated once an epoch of stage N1 sleep occurs, or after 40 minutes if no sleep is recorded
    C. Standard biocalibrations should be performed before each trial
    D. The 20-minute protocol is preferred over the longer 40-minute protocol in assessing an individual's ability to remain awake

101. **Which of the following cardiac rhythm abnormalities is present in this epoch of sleep (see Fig. 8)?**
    A. Sinus tachycardia
    B. Narrow-complex tachycardia
    C. Wide-complex tachycardia
    D. Atrial fibrillation

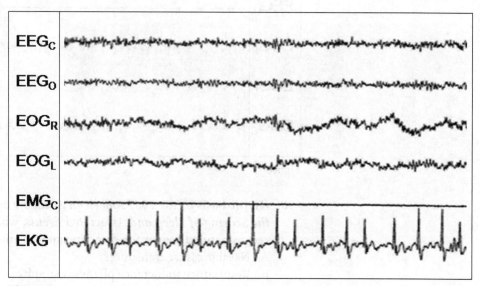

Figure 8.

102. **At what age do electroencephalographic K-complexes start to appear?**
    A. Between 1 and 4 weeks
    B. Between 1 and 2 months
    C. Between 2 and 6 months
    D. After 6 months

103. **Which of the following antidepressants increases REM sleep?**
    A. Amitriptyline
    B. Desipramine
    C. Nefazodone
    D. Protriptyline

104. A 19-year-old college student is evaluated for daytime sleepiness. He reports that his symptoms started 3 years ago during his junior year in high school. He is typically in bed between 11:00 p.m. and 12:30 p.m. on weekdays and at 2:00 a.m. on weekends, but remains awake in bed for at least 60 minutes each night. He awakens after an uneventful evening at 6:00 a.m. on weekdays and between 11:00 a.m. and 11:30 a.m. on weekends. He occasionally takes a 30-minute nap in the late afternoon after returning to his dormitory from school. He describes loud snoring but has not witnessed apneas, restless legs, or cataplexy. He reports occasional episodes of sleep paralysis when he is unable to move for about a minute following awakenings from sleep. He states that he has less difficulty staying up late at night than waking up early in the morning. Indeed, he is generally unable to stay awake during his morning classes and has been late for school many times.

He has a history of exercise-induced asthma. In addition, he was diagnosed with depression a year earlier and has since been taking a selective serotonin reuptake inhibitor. He has tried several over-the-counter sleep aids as well as melatonin with minimal improvement in his sleep latency. In high school, his physician prescribed zolpidem, which he discontinued after 2 weeks as it had no effect on his sleep. He drinks an average of three cans of beer nightly. He also consumes about two cups of coffee each morning. He does not smoke and denies using illicit drugs. Physical examination is unremarkable, and his weight and vital signs are normal.

A 2-week sleep diary was completed by the patient as shown below.

Day	Afternoon						Evening				Midnight		Morning											Noon
	1	2	3	4	5	6	7	8	9	10	11	12	1	2	3	4	5	6	7	8	9	10	11	12
Mon												↓		X	X	X		X	↑					
Tue											↓			X	X	X	X	X	↑					
Wed											↓			X	X	X	X	X	X	↑				
Thu					N							↓		X	X	X	X	↑						
Fri													↓	X	X	X	X	X	X	X	X	↑		
Sat													↓	X	X	X	X	X	X	X	X		↑	
Sun												↓		X	X	X	X	↑						
Mon												↓		X	X	X		X	↑					
Tue			N									↓		X	X	X	X	X	X	↑				
Wed												↓		X	X	X	X	X	↑					
Thu									N			↓		X	X	X	X	↑						
Fri													↓		X	X	X	X	X	X	X	↑		
Sat												↓		X	X	X	X	X	X	X	↑			
Sun												↓		X	X	X	X	↑						

↓, bedtime; ↑, time out of bed; X, sleep; N, naps.

Which of the following would be the most appropriate management for this patient?
A. Bright light exposure during the morning before the core body temperature nadir (CTmin)
B. Bright light exposure during the morning after the CTmin
C. Bright light exposure during the evening before the CTmin
D. Bright light exposure during the evening after the CTmin

105. **Which of the following statements concerning jet lag is true?**
A. The severity of jet lag symptoms is directly related to the amount of time zone transitions but not to the direction of travel
B. Individuals commonly complain of sleep initiation insomnia following westward flights and early morning awakenings after eastward travel
C. Jet lag symptoms generally persist longer following westward travel
D. Evening exposure to bright light after westward travel and morning exposure after eastward travel can hasten synchronization to the new time zone

106. **At what age does a child typically develop the ability to sleep through the night (i.e., nocturnal sleep consolidation)?**
A. Between 3 and 6 months
B. Between 6 and 9 months
C. Between 9 and 12 months
D. Between 12 and 15 months

107. **According to the Speilman theory regarding the pathogenesis of insomnia, which of the following is considered a predisposing factor for sleep disturbance?**
A. Maladaptive sleep–wake behaviors
B. Physiologic hyperarousal
C. Alterations in sleep–wake schedules
D. Poor sleep hygiene

108. **Which of the following behavioral therapies for insomnia involves increasing homeostatic sleep drive by reducing time in bed and matching the latter with the actual duration of total sleep time?**
A. Paradoxical intention
B. Sleep restriction
C. Stimulus control
D. Temporal control

109. **Which of the following clinical features best describes psychophysiologic insomnia?**
A. Anxiety is not limited to sleep, but pervades other areas of daily living
B. Sleep disturbance is directly related to an identifiable stressor and sleep generally improves with resolution of the stressor
C. Sleep quality is always worse in the sleep laboratory compared to the patient's usual sleep at home (i.e., first-night effect)
D. It tends to affect women more than men

110. **Which of the following pathogens is responsible for sleeping sickness?**
    A. Cyclospora
    B. Schistosoma
    C. Toxoplasma
    D. Trypanosoma

111. **Which of the following clinical features best describes narcolepsy without cataplexy?**
    A. Absence of sleep paralysis and hypnagogic hallucinations
    B. Cataplexy-like symptoms can be present
    C. Low levels of cerebrospinal fluid (CSF) hypocretin-1 in most patients
    D. Accounts for less than 5% of cases of narcolepsy

112. **Which of the following statements regarding the differences between narcolepsy and idiopathic hypersomnia is true?**
    A. Daytime naps are transiently refreshing in narcolepsy but sleepiness tends to persist despite napping in patients with idiopathic hypersomnia
    B. Sleep-onset REM periods during multiple sleep latency testing are more common in patients with idiopathic hypersomnia compared to those with narcolepsy
    C. HLA CW2 positivity is more likely to be present in patients with narcolepsy than in patients with idiopathic hypersomnia
    D. Sleepiness in patients with idiopathic hypersomnia responds better and more predictably to stimulant therapy than in those with narcolepsy

113. **Which of the following statements regarding human leukocyte antigen (HLA) typing in narcolepsy is true?**
    A. A negative test for DQB1*0602 does not exclude the diagnosis of narcolepsy, since an estimated 1% to 5% of all narcoleptics are negative for this HLA type
    B. The prevalence of DR2 is higher among African American patients with narcolepsy compared to Caucasians with the similar disorder
    C. Most multiplex family cases (i.e., multiple members of the family with narcolepsy) are HLA DQB1*0602 negative
    D. HLA DQB1*0602 positivity is more common in patients with narcolepsy without cataplexy than in those with cataplexy

114. **Which of the following statements best describes the differences between nightmares and sleep terrors?**
    A. Nightmares generally occur during the latter half of the night, whereas sleep terrors occur earlier during the first half of the nocturnal sleep period
    B. Nightmares emerge during REM sleep, while sleep terrors arise from stage N1 sleep
    C. Persons are often confused and disoriented following awakenings from nightmares, but are awake and alert with sleep terrors
    D. Subsequent return to sleep is rapid following nightmares and delayed with sleep terrors

115. **What is the estimated annual spontaneous cure rate in children with primary sleep enuresis?**
   A. 5%
   B. 10%
   C. 15%
   D. 20%

116. **Which of the following factors has been shown to increase the risk of developing periodic breathing secondary to high altitude?**
   A. REM sleep
   B. Decreased hypoxic ventilatory chemoresponsiveness
   C. Female gender
   D. Rapid ascent

117. **Which of the following statements regarding the pathogenesis of nocturnal asthma is correct?**
   A. Airflow displays a circadian variability and is highest in the early morning
   B. Functional residual capacity is greater during sleep compared to wakefulness
   C. Snoring and obstructive sleep apnea contribute to upper airway obstruction
   D. Bronchospasm is exacerbated by the relative reduction in parasympathetic tone during sleep compared to waking levels

118. **Which of the following statements about sleep in patients with human immunodeficiency virus (HIV) infection is true?**
   A. Patients with HIV disease generally have no objective changes in polysomnographic parameters despite subjective complaints of significant sleep disruption
   B. The antiviral therapy, efavirenz, is frequently associated with sedation and excessive sleepiness
   C. Zidovudine can cause sleep disturbance and insomnia
   D. Sleep quality is not influenced by the underlying immune status (e.g., T cell counts)

119. **Which of the following statements describes the differences between childhood and adult obstructive sleep apnea?**
   A. Excessive sleepiness is more common in children than among adults
   B. Whereas it is more prevalent in adult men, there is no gender difference in children
   C. Oxygen desaturation related to respiratory events is more pronounced in children compared to adult patients
   D. Changes in sleep architecture, including a decrease in stage N3, are more likely to be seen in children than in adults

120. A 4-year-old boy is brought to you by his mother for management of persistent insomnia of 12-month duration. The patient typically has dinner at 7:00 p.m. and then spends an hour either watching television or playing with his two older brothers, who are 7 and 10 years of age. He is then brought to his bedroom by his father at 8:30 p.m. but frequently walks out to get a drink of water after only a few minutes. He may ask to be read to in bed, or may go to the family room to join his brothers in watching television. His father then has to bring him back to his bedroom, only to have him leave his bedroom again; this may be repeated several times during the night. He admits to you that he is not scared of being alone in his bedroom. Interestingly, 2 months ago, when his grandparents came to visit them for a few days, he had no difficulty falling asleep on his own when all three of the children were firmly and steadfastly asked to go to bed at their customary bedtime.

   He is healthy with no medical illnesses and currently takes no medications. His pediatrician had recommended a trial of diphenhydramine to help with his sleep but his mother is uneasy about giving him this medication. He attends a half-day kindergarten class three times a week, which he seems to enjoy doing. He is physically active and is a member of his local community swim team in his age group. According to his mother, none of his older brothers ever had difficulty falling asleep when they were younger.

   Which of the following causes of childhood insomnia is the most likely diagnosis?
   A. Limit-setting sleep disorder
   B. Psychophysiologic insomnia
   C. Sleep-onset association disorder
   D. Delayed sleep phase syndrome

121. According to Bonnet's classic studies on sleep fragmentation, which of the following statements regarding sleep fragmentation is correct?
   A. At least 10 to 20 minutes of consolidated sleep is required for normal restorative effect
   B. Daytime sleepiness is more closely related to sleep stage deprivation than to sleep fragmentation
   C. Total sleep deprivation has a much greater impact on multiple sleep latency test (MSLT) scores than frequent (every 1 to 2 minutes) but brief electroencephalographic arousals
   D. Sleep fragmentation negatively affects performance but has little effect on hormones or respiratory parameters

122. Actigraphy is often used in sleep medicine to obtain an estimate of sleep. Which of the following statements about actigraphy is true?
   A. Is less reliable than a sleep log in determining brief arousals from sleep
   B. May overestimate sleep time in depressed patients who remain motionless while awake
   C. Has little utility in shift work since it does not provide any measure of core temperature
   D. Is often expensive and technically difficult to administer and therefore may not be appropriate for elderly or demented patients

123. **In patients with gastroesophageal reflux disease (GERD), when does the majority of reflux events occur?**
    A. N2 sleep
    B. N1 sleep
    C. During awakenings from sleep
    D. REM sleep

124. **Unlike dreaming in normal individuals, the dreams of individuals with posttraumatic stress disorder (PTSD):**
    A. Typically arise during stage N3 sleep
    B. Often incorporate actual memories of frightening experiences
    C. Are more easily recalled
    D. Often lack atonia

125. **A 39-year-old woman completes a sleep study. She is taking at least one medication. On the basis of the sleep architecture below, what is the most likely medication that she is taking?**

Stage 1—1.4%

Stage 2—67%

Stage 3—22%

Stage REM—9.2%

Sleep Onset Latency—17 minutes

REM Latency—303 minutes

    A. Benzodiazepine
    B. Non-benzodiazepine hypnotic agent
    C. Antidepressant
    D. Oral contraceptive

126. **Longitudinal and population-based studies on the relationship between insomnia and mood disorders have shown which of the following clinical features?**
    A. Insomnia alone does not confer an increased risk for subsequent development of a new-onset psychiatric illness
    B. Insomnia is best thought of as a symptom that is secondary to depression or anxiety
    C. Effective treatment of an underlying mental illness will result in significant improvements in sleep
    D. Insomnia can often predict relapse of a mood disorder

127. **Sleep restriction therapy for the treatment of chronic insomnia theoretically improves sleep by which of the following?**
    A. By increasing homeostatic sleep drive
    B. By realigning the circadian sleep phase to more closely correlate with minimum body temperature
    C. Through paradoxical avoidance of performance anxiety (i.e., "I must sleep")
    D. By decreasing negative associations between the bedroom and sleep

128. **The acute effects of alcohol on sleep in nonalcoholics include which of the following?**
    A. Acute use of alcohol can decrease sleep-onset latency and increase both stage N3 and REM sleep during the first portion of the night
    B. Alcohol selectively decreases muscle tone in the upper airway, leading to the development or worsening of both snoring and obstructive sleep apnea
    C. Once alcohol is metabolized, often halfway through the night, sleep appears to be normal for the remainder of the night
    D. Daytime alcohol consumption causes less impairment in a sleep-deprived individual than in one who is well rested

129. **A 62-year-old man has been abstinent from alcohol for 8 months. He continues to complain of difficulty falling and staying asleep. Polysomnography failed to reveal any sleep-disordered breathing or periodic limb movements during sleep. He has very little stage N3 sleep and has a shortened REM latency. Which of the following statements is true?**
    A. It is unlikely that past alcohol abuse continues to exert a negative effect on sleep after so much time without alcohol
    B. The insomnia complaint makes it more likely that he will relapse within a year
    C. Because of cross-tolerance, it is unlikely that benzodiazepines would improve his sleep
    D. The sleep changes suggest that he may be abusing another drug besides alcohol

130. **This is a diagnostic hypnogram of a 52-year-old man with complaints of loud snoring and excessive daytime sleepiness. He denies sleep paralysis, hypnagogic hallucination, or cataplexy. The only medication he is taking is diclofenac. However, he had discontinued desipramine 1 week prior to the sleep study. Polysomnography shows an apnea–hypopnea index (AHI) of 12. All episodes are hypopneas and the nadir oxygen saturation is 91%. Sleep efficiency is 85%, with 9% N1 stage, 39% N2, 0% N3 sleep, and 52% REM sleep. REM latency from sleep onset is 32 minutes, but removing intervening wake time, it was 8 minutes. How would you interpret this hypnogram?**
    A. The study shows mild sleep apnea but is otherwise a normal sleep study
    B. The sleep architecture suggests a diagnosis of narcolepsy
    C. The sleep architecture suggests a diagnosis of depression
    D. The sleep architecture suggests a medication effect

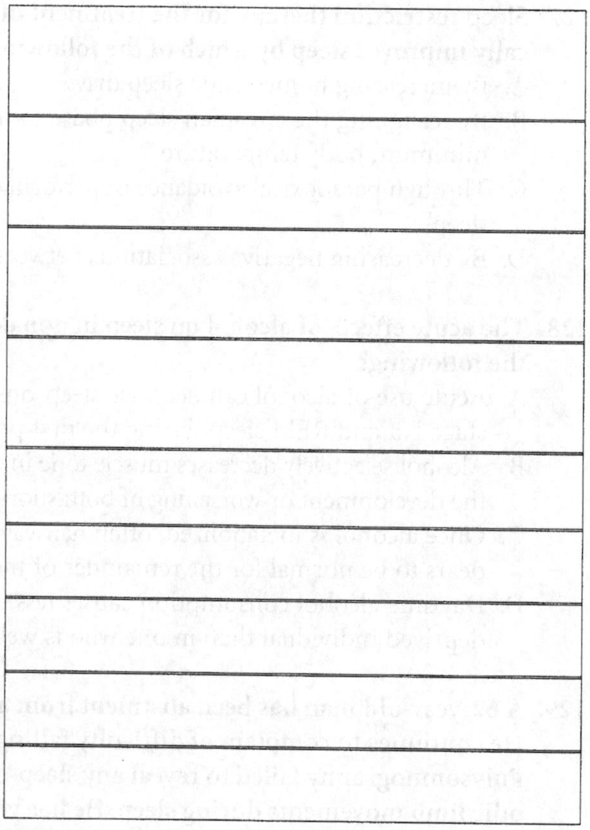

Figure 9.

131. The phase response curve (PRC) characterizes the effects of stimuli on the circadian pacemaker. Both light and melatonin have distinctive PRCs. A 16-year-old boy has a 3-year history of being unable to fall asleep until 2:00 a.m. and sleeping until spontaneously awakening at 11:00 a.m. His school schedule requires that he gets up at 7:00 a.m. and he therefore needs to be asleep much earlier than his current 2:00 a.m. How would you best phase shift this young man's circadian sleep–wake rhythm?
   A. Phase advance with evening bright light exposure and morning melatonin administration
   B. Phase advance with evening melatonin administration and morning bright light exposure
   C. Phase advance with evening melatonin administration and evening bright light exposure
   D. Phase delay with evening bright light exposure and morning melatonin administration

132. **What is the primary use of the constant routine protocol?**
   A. A behavioral technique to improve sleep habits for the treatment of insomnia
   B. A forced relaxation test to quantify severity of restless legs syndrome
   C. A monitoring technique used to assess circadian rhythms
   D. A monitoring technique used in conjunction with actigraphy to assess long-term sleep habits

133. **Ekbom, in 1960, noted that restless legs syndrome (RLS) occurs commonly in patients with iron deficiency anemia. What is the theoretical association between iron and RLS?**
    A. Low iron levels interfere with gamma aminobutyric acid (GABA) transmission
    B. Iron is a cofactor for tyrosine hydroxylase, the rate-limiting enzyme in dopamine synthesis
    C. Magnetic resonance imaging (MRI) studies show decreased levels of iron in the motor cortex of persons with RLS compared to age-matched control subjects
    D. More recent investigations have failed to show any significant correlation between iron status and RLS

134. **The intrinsic circadian sleep–wake rhythm in humans does not run at exactly 24 hours. Synchronization with the 24-hour day depends on exposure to environmental time signals. Which of the following statements is correct?**
    A. Functional rods and cones are necessary for light entrainment to occur
    B. Nonphotic time cues (e.g., scheduled sleep and activity, exercise, or meals) are as important as the solar light–dark cycle in maintaining the circadian system
    C. Although full spectrum lights are often used, blue wavelength light is more efficient than full spectrum light in shifting the circadian system
    D. Light intensity of less than 1,000 lux has almost no effect on circadian rhythms

135. **Seventy-one percent of menstruating women report that their sleep is affected by menstrual symptoms a few days each month. Which of the following is an objective finding regarding sleep across the menstrual cycle?**
    A. Thermogenic action of progesterone secreted from the corpus luteum causes a slight increase in core body temperature and a greater nocturnal decline in body temperature
    B. Sleep-onset latency and sleep efficiency show more changes in the luteal phase compared to the follicular phase
    C. Women have a shorter REM latency as well as a small decrease in REM sleep in the luteal phase compared to the follicular phase
    D. Women taking oral contraceptives have elevated body temperatures that fall back to normal levels during the placebo period of the oral contraceptive pack

136. **Jet lag occurs when rapid travel across time zones leads to a mismatch between the internal circadian rhythms and local time cues. The internal circadian sleep–wake rhythm can adapt but does so slowly. Which of the following statements regarding jet lag is accurate?**
    A. Travel in an eastward direction takes longer to adapt to and is often seen as difficulty falling asleep and more wakefulness early in the night
    B. Travel in a westward direction takes longer to adapt to and may show good-quality sleep early in the night with increased REM sleep and awakenings toward early morning

    C. Adaptation to the new time zone is determined by the number of time zones crossed rather than the direction traveled

    D. Most countermeasures including light exposure, hypnotics, and melatonin have not been shown to substantially improve jet lag

137. **The multiple sleep latency test (MSLT) is used to objectively determine the level of sleepiness and to help make the diagnosis of narcolepsy. Using a clinical protocol, what are the shortest and longest times that any individual nap opportunity could be conducted?**
    A. 1.5 minutes and 20 minutes
    B. 15 minutes and 35 minutes
    C. 15 minutes and 20 minutes
    D. The test always lasts 20 minutes

138. **A 30-year-old gentleman has a 5-year history of difficulty falling asleep and staying asleep during the night. He consumes five cups of coffee each day, all before 6:00 p.m., and gets in bed at 9:00 p.m. but is usually awake until 1:00 a.m. He watches television in bed and often leaves the set on all night. There is a clock by his bed and he frequently checks the time during the night, particularly during the multiple awakenings in the night. He awakens spontaneously at 8:00 a.m. He reports variability in his sleep time but believes that he is getting about 6 hours of sleep per night. Polysomnography finds no evidence of snoring, obstructive sleep apnea, or periodic limb movements during sleep. He has several awakenings that are scored as spontaneous arousals. It took him 56 minutes to fall asleep after turning the lights out at 10:00 p.m. He was awakened in the sleep laboratory at 6:00 a.m. His total sleep time is 6.5 hours with normal sleep stage percentages and sleep architecture. He takes no medications. He is somewhat "high strung" and he describes that his "mind is very active at night." He denies significant anxiety or depression. He reports that his sleep in the sleep laboratory was similar to that at home. He does not typically sleep any better or worse when away from home. He occasionally has a good night of sleep once he "gets exhausted" from several nights of little or no sleep. He has never taken a medication for sleep and is afraid of getting addicted to sleeping pills.**

    On the basis of your understanding of behavioral interventions for insomnia, if you could use only one therapy, which of the following would you choose?
    A. Sleep hygiene therapy
    B. Relaxation therapy
    C. Stimulus control therapy
    D. Sleep restriction therapy

139. **There is a substantial increase in sleep complaints during menopause. The current research on sleep during menopause shows which of the following?**
    A. Apart from sleep disturbance caused by hot flashes, objective polysomnographic measures do not show significant sleep changes consistent with subjective complaints
    B. Both subjective and objective measures show clear disruption of sleep with an increase in sleep-onset latency and decrease in sleep efficiency

C. Hormone replacement therapy has a substantial impact on both objective and subjective sleep measures, even in women who experience mild or infrequent hot flashes

D. Hot flashes typically end within a year or two of the last menstrual period

140. **According to the activation-synthesis theory of dreaming, dreams differ from normal consciousness primarily because of which of the following?**
A. The chemical control of the brain in the two states is entirely different
B. Repressed psychologic issues are more readily accessible during sleep, particularly in REM sleep
C. Dreams have a much higher affective component than waking thought
D. Dreams make much broader connections than waking thoughts and, as a result, have a more calming effect

141. **Both ambient and body temperatures can influence sleep. Studies examining the effects of temperature on sleep have found which of the following?**
A. Stage N3 sleep increases in cooler temperatures relative to thermoneutrality (29°C) and decreases in warmer temperatures
B. REM sleep is less sensitive than NREM sleep to ambient temperature changes, probably due to the loss of thermoregulatory processes in NREM sleep
C. Both passive heating and high-intensity exercise increase stage N3 sleep
D. Sleep effects seen with temperature changes are more strongly related to the rate of fall of body temperature rather than to the body temperature itself

142. **A 45-year-old man comes to your office complaining of sleepiness. He is tired throughout the day. He goes to bed at midnight, falls asleep easily, sleeps soundly, and awakens daily at 5:30 a.m. to get ready for work. He does not snore or have any witnessed apneic episodes. He is chronically sleepy and drinks caffeine in the morning and at noon to stay awake. If he drinks any caffeine after lunch, he has difficulty falling asleep at night. He feels he could nap during the day but does not have any time for it. He sleeps until 6:30 a.m. on the weekends but feels no better. What would be your first recommendation?**
A. Take melatonin in the evening and use light therapy in the morning
B. Obtain a sleep study looking for sleep-disordered breathing
C. Encourage him to try to get more sleep each night
D. Encourage him to decrease his caffeine use

143. **A 63-year-old woman is referred to you because of uncontrolled hypertension. Her physician has tried various antihypertensive agents without success. She is obese and states that others have complained of her snoring though she sleeps well at night. She undergoes a polysomnogram and is found to have severe obstructive sleep apnea. Which of the following statements regarding changes in blood pressure during sleep is true?**
A. Surge in blood pressure occurs immediately before an apneic episode
B. Surge in blood pressure usually occurs during the apneic episode
C. Surge in blood pressure usually occurs immediately after an apneic episode
D. There is no relationship between surge in blood pressure and apnea

144. **Which of the following statements about the relationship between subjective complaints of sleepiness as measured by sleepiness scales, such as the Epworth Sleepiness Scale, and severity of obstructive sleep apnea as determined by the apnea–hypopnea index is true?**
   A. There is a direct linear correlation between severity of obstructive sleep apnea and the Epworth Sleepiness Scale
   B. Only about half of patients with moderate to severe obstructive sleep apnea will complain of excessive daytime sleepiness
   C. Obstructive sleep apnea does not warrant treatment if a patient does not complain of excessive daytime sleepiness
   D. A patient with severe obstructive sleep apnea will complain of more severe sleepiness than a patient with mild obstructive sleep apnea

145. **What wavelength of light is most effective for phototherapy in delayed sleep phase syndrome?**
   A. Polychromatic (white) light
   B. Monochromatic "yellow" light of about 580 nm
   C. Monochromatic "blue" light of about 460 nm
   D. Monochromatic "green" light of about 555 nm

146. **What does the following epoch (see Fig. 10) demonstrate?**
   A. Seizure activity
   B. Bruxism
   C. Alpha intrusion
   D. Hypnic jerk

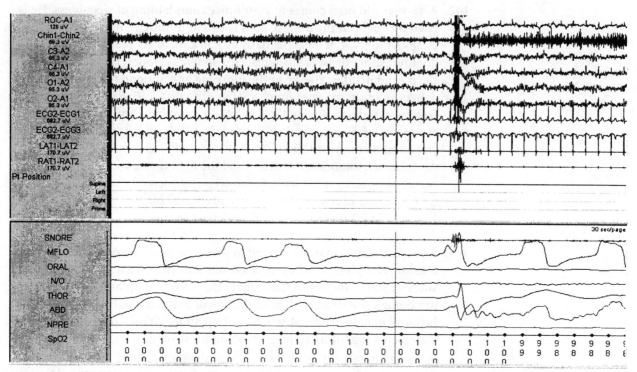

Figure 10.

147. **How do first-generation antihistamines affect sleep architecture?**
   A. Decrease REM sleep
   B. Decrease stage N2 sleep
   C. Increase stage N2 sleep
   D. Increase REM sleep

148. **A child is being evaluated for attention deficit hyperactivity disorder. His mother states that he has been a poor sleeper all his life. Despite this, he seems inattentive and hyperactive rather than sleepy during the day. What would you recommend for her son?**
   A. Start a stimulant
   B. Refer to an otolaryngologist for adenotonsillectomy
   C. Recommend melatonin therapy
   D. Perform a polysomnography

149. **Which statement regarding pseudo-spindles observed during sleep is true?**
   A. Represent an arousal–sleep pattern associated with sleepiness
   B. Seen in patients taking tricyclic antidepressants
   C. Common in patients with fibromyalgia
   D. Usually slightly faster in frequency than sleep spindles

150. **A 39-year-old man moved from San Francisco, California, to Denver, Colorado, about 2 months ago. He was diagnosed with obstructive sleep apnea (OSA) 2 years ago when he presented with severe snoring and daytime sleepiness. This was treated with positive airway pressure therapy that is set at a pressure of 10 cm H_2O. He now complains of a return of daytime sleepiness since the move. Which of the following has likely occurred with regard to his OSA?**
   A. He has developed central sleep apnea in addition to his OSA as a result of the move
   B. His obstructive apneic events have increased significantly as a result of the move
   C. His OSA has not changed but he is stressed from the move
   D. His continuous positive airway pressure (CPAP) machine is not working as a result of the elevation change

151. **What is the first-line treatment for a child with obstructive sleep apnea?**
   A. Weight loss
   B. Adenotonsillectomy
   C. Positive airway pressure therapy
   D. Iron supplementation

152. **In the 5-minute polysomnographic tracing shown in Figure 11, which statement regarding the respiratory pattern seen is correct?**
   A. It represents paradoxical respiratory effort seen in obstructive sleep apnea
   B. It tends to be worse during NREM sleep and resolves during REM sleep
   C. It tends to be worse during REM sleep and resolves during REM sleep
   D. It tends to be worse during nonsupine sleep

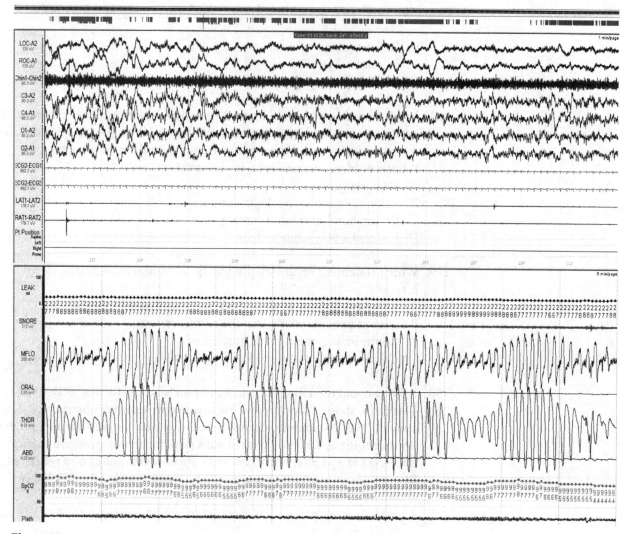

Figure 11.

153. Which of the following statements regarding nocturnal enuresis is correct?
A. New-onset enuresis in adults is not associated with obstructive sleep apnea
B. It is more common in children with sleep-disordered breathing than in healthy children
C. It is a behavioral condition and is not related to sleep-disordered breathing
D. It occurs because of an increase in nocturnal antidiuretic hormone (ADH)

154. Which statement regarding the effect of nicotine use on sleep is true?
A. Nicotine decreases sleep latency and improves sleep quality
B. Nicotine decreases nighttime arousals
C. Withdrawal symptoms include increased alertness during the day
D. Withdrawal symptoms include increased nocturnal arousals

155. **Which of the following statements regarding compliance to therapy in obstructive sleep apnea is true?**
    A. Bi-level positive airway pressure improves compliance in unselected patients
    B. Auto-titrating continuous positive airway therapy improves compliance
    C. Heated humidity improves compliance
    D. Flexible continuous positive airway pressure (CPAP) (CFlex) does not improve compliance

156. **Which statement best describes the abnormality seen in the electroencephalogram leads in Figure 12?**
    A. It represents a "spike-and-wave" abnormality
    B. It is snore artifact
    C. It is a result of a poor M2 electrode
    D. It is artifact from the electrocardiogram

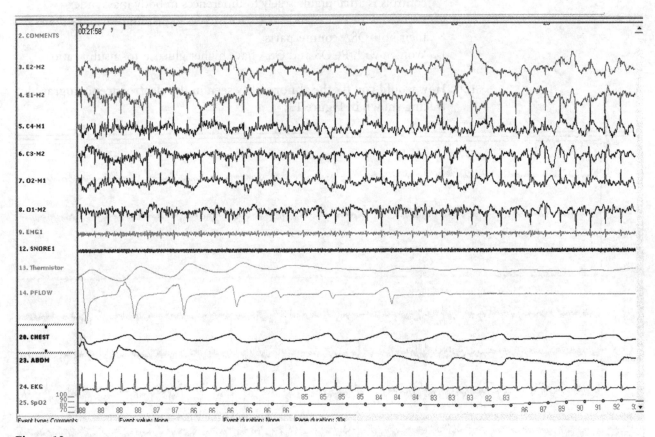

Figure 12.

157. **Which statement is correct regarding chronic renal failure patients with sleep apnea?**
    A. Renal transplantation has not been shown to affect central or obstructive sleep apneas
    B. Nocturnal hemodialysis decreases central and obstructive apneas
    C. A minority of chronic renal failure patients have been shown to have obstructive sleep apnea
    D. Patients with chronic renal failure tend to be hypercapnic

158. **Which of the following statements regarding modafinil is true?**
    A. It is hepatically cleared and requires dose adjustments in hepatic impairment
    B. It has been shown to effectively treat cataplexy
    C. Peak concentration is achieved in 6 to 8 hours
    D. There is no associated cardiovascular risk with long-term use

159. **Women with polycystic ovarian syndrome (PCOS) have a higher prevalence of obstructive sleep apnea (OSA) than their premenopausal counterparts. However, not all patients with PCOS have OSA. Which of the following statements may explain the factors involved in the development of OSA in these patients?**
    A. PCOS patients with OSA have lower testosterone levels than their non-OSA counterparts
    B. The difference between PCOS patients with OSA versus age-matched controls is attributable solely to differences in body mass index
    C. Women with PCOS and OSA have increased insulin resistance than their non-OSA counterparts
    D. Women with PCOS and OSA have higher glucose-to-insulin ratios

160. **How would you fix the abnormality seen in the electroencephalographic tracing shown in Figure 13?**

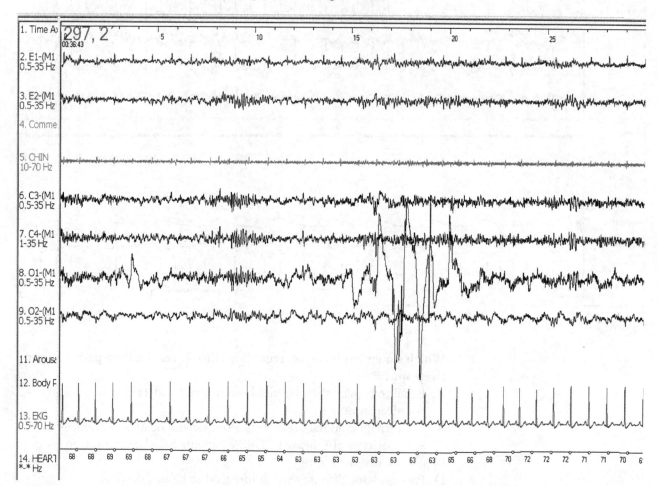

Figure 13.

A. Immediately administer lorazepam intravenously
B. Change to a low-pass filter in the O1-M1 lead
C. Reapply the O1 electrode
D. Turn on a fan and cool the room

161. **Which of the following statements regarding periodic limb movements (PLMs) and restless legs syndrome (RLS) is true?**
    A. About 80% of patients with RLS have PLMs
    B. About 80% of patients with PLMs have RLS
    C. There is no relationship between PLMs and RLS
    D. Both PLMs and RLS require polysomnography for diagnosis

162. **Which of the following statements regarding gamma hydroxybutyrate (GHB) used for narcolepsy is correct?**
    A. Exacerbates cataplexy
    B. Increases slow-wave sleep
    C. Increases nocturnal arousals
    D. Much of its effect is via stimulation of serotonin receptors

163. **Which of the following would be observed after acute sleep deprivation in a 25-year-old person?**
    A. Increase in REM sleep
    B. Increase in N3 sleep
    C. Increase in N1 sleep
    D. Increase in N2 sleep

164. **Which of the following statements regarding nocturnal seizures is correct?**
    A. Seizure threshold is lower during NREM sleep
    B. Seizure threshold is lower during REM sleep
    C. Seizure threshold is higher during sleep deprivation
    D. Nocturnal seizures do not contribute to daytime sleepiness

165. **Which of the following statements regarding prolactin secretion is correct?**
    A. Has its own circadian rhythm which is not influenced by sleep state
    B. Closely associated with sleep onset
    C. Increases after nocturnal sleep periods but not during daytime sleep onset
    D. Increases immediately before arousal from sleep

166. **Which of the following statements regarding the prevalence of sleep-disordered breathing in the US population is correct?**
    A. The estimated prevalence in middle-aged men is 5%
    B. About 10% of middle-aged adults screen high for a risk of obstructive sleep apnea
    C. About 80% of middle-aged adults screen high for a risk of obstructive sleep apnea
    D. The estimated prevalence in middle-aged men is 40%

167. A 73-year-old man develops tremors of the extremities, rigidity, and slow movements. He is diagnosed with Parkinson disease (PD) by a neurologist and is treated with pramipexole. Subsequently, the patient develops symptoms of excessive daytime sleepiness (EDS) and is referred for a sleep consultation. Which of the following is correct in the assessment of EDS in patients with PD?
    A. A complaint of EDS usually occurs early in the course of PD and in younger patients
    B. Dopaminergic medications have a mildly stimulating property, and treatment with dopaminergic medications results in improvement in EDS
    C. Dopaminergic drugs are associated with complaints of excessive daytime sleepiness
    D. Amphetamines are the only effective medications for treating excessive sleepiness in PD

168. Which of the following is true regarding the relationship between obstructive sleep apnea (OSA) and stroke?
    A. The increased risk of stroke seen in patients with OSA is mainly accounted for by the presence of atrial fibrillation in these patients
    B. The increased risk of OSA in patients with stroke is most likely due to the presence of pharyngeal dysfunction in patients who have suffered a stroke
    C. The association of stroke and OSA has been shown to be caused by the presence of a patent foramen ovale in these patients
    D. The presence of OSA has been shown to be a significant risk factor in stroke, independent of other risk factors such as hypertension, hyperlipidemia, atrial fibrillation, and diabetes

169. Which of the following neurodegenerative diseases has not been shown to be associated with REM sleep behavior disorder (RBD)?
    A. Alzheimer disease
    B. Multisystem atrophy
    C. Lewy body dementia
    D. Parkinson disease

170. Which of the following tests is most helpful in guiding therapy for a patient with restless legs syndrome (RLS)?
    A. Serum calcium level over 11.0 mg/dL
    B. Serum iron level less than 110 μg/dL
    C. Serum total iron-binding capacity greater than 400 μg/dL
    D. Serum ferritin level less than 50 μg/L

171. Which of the following neurotransmitters is abnormally low or absent in the brain of patients with narcolepsy?
    A. Acetylcholine
    B. Norepinephrine
    C. Hypocretin
    D. Gamma aminobutyric acid (GABA)

172. **The CLOCK gene plays an important role in regulating circadian rhythms. Which of the following best describes its function?**
    A. The CLOCK gene encodes for a protein that is found exclusively in the retina adjacent to rods and cones that responds to changes in light
    B. CLOCK-related mRNA is found exclusively in the suprachiasmatic nucleus (SCN) and the retinohypothalamic tract and not in other tissues
    C. CLOCK gene–related protein is the only protein identified so far that has significant influences on circadian rhythm
    D. Delayed sleep phase syndrome, in some families, has an autosomal dominant mode of inheritance and is associated with polymorphisms of the CLOCK gene

173. **Compared to wakefulness, which of the following is true regarding ventilation during REM sleep in a normal person?**
    A. Ventilatory response to $PaCO_2$ is markedly reduced
    B. Ventilatory response to PaO_2 increases leading to more frequent central apneas
    C. Intercostal muscles assume a larger role in ventilation
    D. Responsiveness to $PaCO_2$ increases in women compared to men

174. **Which of the following is classified as a wakefulness-promoting neurotransmitter?**
    A. Histamine
    B. Serotonin
    C. Gamma aminobutyric acid (GABA)
    D. Adenosine

175. **Which of the following statements regarding the effects of melatonin administration on circadian rhythms is most accurate?**
    A. Phase response effect for melatonin is identical to that for administered bright light
    B. Melatonin administered 6 hours after the core body temperature minimum will phase advance the circadian rhythm
    C. Melatonin administered 6 hours before the core body temperature minimum will phase delay the circadian rhythm
    D. Melatonin administered 6 hours before the core body temperature minimum will phase advance the circadian rhythm

176. **A 52-year-old woman is referred for evaluation of nonrefreshing and nonrestorative sleep. She has severe kyphoscoliosis and is markedly debilitated. She reports going to bed at 10:00 p.m. but takes at least 45 to 60 minutes to fall asleep. She has multiple awakenings during the night and awakens earlier than she would like to at 4:00 a.m. to 5:00 a.m. Pulmonary function studies show that total lung capacity is reduced to 64% of predicted and vital capacity is 54% of predicted. FEV_1 is 0.8 L and the FEV_1/FVC ratio is 0.80. Arterial blood gases show a PaO_2 of 56 mm Hg, $PaCO_2$ of 58 mm Hg, pH 7.38, and serum bicarbonate level of 34 mEq/L.**

    Polysomnography is performed. Total sleep time is 4.3 hours and sleep efficiency is 48%. There is 20% stage N1 sleep, 68% stage N2 sleep,

2% stage N3 sleep, and 10% stage R sleep. Apnea–hypopnea index (AHI) is 24 events per hour and the central apnea index is 10 per hour. Sixty percent of oximetry recordings are below 90%, and SaO_2 decreases to 58% during stage R sleep. Which of the following is the most appropriate treatment of her sleep problem?
A. Zolpidem 5 mg orally 3 hours before sleep and increasing to 10 mg if there is no response
B. Supplemental oxygen at 2 to 3 L/min
C. Noninvasive positive airway pressure at settings established during a second-night polysomnography
D. Nasal continuous positive airway pressure (CPAP) set at a pressure established during a second-night polysomnography

177. Stage N3 sleep is characterized by which of the following electroencephalographic criteria?
A. Scored when 20% or more of the epoch consists of deflections of 0.5 to 2.0 Hz frequency and >75 mV of amplitude
B. Scored when 50% or more of the epoch consists of deflections of 0.5 to 2.0 Hz frequency and >75 mV of amplitude
C. Scored when 20% or more of the epoch consists of deflections of 0.5 to 2.0 Hz frequency and >75 mV of amplitude in children or amplitude >50 mV in adults and the elderly
D. Scored when 50% or more of the epoch consists of deflections of 2.0 to 5.0 Hz frequency and >75 mV of amplitude

178. REM sleep is characterized by atonia of skeletal muscles. Which neurotransmitter is released in the spinal column motoneurons and appears to be responsible for the atonia associated with REM sleep?
A. Dopamine
B. Hypocretin
C. Glycine
D. Norepinephrine

179. Gamma hydroxybutyrate (GHB, sodium oxybate) is effective for which of the following sleep disorders?
A. Restless legs syndrome
B. REM behavior disorder
C. Narcolepsy with cataplexy
D. Delayed sleep phase syndrome

180. A low-frequency filter that is set at 5 Hz would be expected to have which effect on the electroencephalogram with relationship to monitoring sleep stages?
A. This filter setting would eliminate the artifact related to excessive sweat
B. This filter setting would eliminate 60-Hz artifact
C. This filter setting would enhance delta waves, making stage N3 sleep easier to identify
D. This filter setting would make the identification of N2 sleep more difficult by suppressing sleep spindles

181. A 54-year-old woman seeks consultation regarding long-standing trouble with her sleep. She has been using lorazepam 2 mg at bedtime for many years. She had a prior polysomnogram that showed no evidence of obstructive sleep apnea, but demonstrated prolonged sleep latency and low sleep efficiency. She has no history of depression and a psychiatric consultation reveals no clinical signs of depression or other psychiatric illness. Her primary care physician would like her to stop the use of lorazepam, but she has been very resistant to this. She reports that she does not sleep at all if she does not take lorazepam at bedtime and is concerned that her sleep problem will only get worse without the drug. She is experiencing mild difficulty with memory and concentration and is more forgetful about important things than she had been in the past. What is the most appropriate action to take at this time?
    A. Advise her to continue lorazepam
    B. Refer her for drug addiction counseling
    C. Discuss the possibility of rebound insomnia and provide instructions in sleep hygiene, cognitive behavioral therapy, and drug taper
    D. Prescribe a tricyclic antidepressant at bedtime and discontinue her lorazepam

182. Which of the following hypnotic drugs acts primarily on the melatonin receptors in the brain and has little affinity for benzodiazepine receptors?
    A. Eszopiclone
    B. Temazepam
    C. Trazodone
    D. Ramelteon

183. Which of the following symptoms has the highest diagnostic value in making the clinical diagnosis of narcolepsy?
    A. Hypnagogic hallucinations
    B. Excessive daytime sleepiness
    C. Restless legs during sleep
    D. Cataplexy

184. A 19-year-old woman sees you in consultation for evaluation of excessive daytime sleepiness. She has experienced profound sleepiness for several years and she has fallen asleep in school several times. If she takes a nap, she feels refreshed for several hours, but invariably sleepiness recurs. She has noted an unusual sensation of weakness in her legs and finds she has to hold onto a chair or table to maintain her balance when she laughs at a humorous story. A polysomnogram showed 7.2 hours of sleep and no evidence of sleep-disordered breathing. A multiple sleep latency test showed a mean sleep latency of 4.3 minutes and two naps with REM sleep. Which of the following drugs is indicated for this individual's condition?
    A. Lamictal
    B. Pramipexole
    C. Modafinil
    D. Pregalbin

185. A 34-year-old man seeks your consultation for a complaint of insomnia. He describes insomnia dating back to his high school years. He goes to bed at approximately 10:00 p.m. but is unable to fall asleep for 3 to 4 hours. He finally falls asleep at about 1:00 a.m. to 2:00 a.m. and then sleeps soundly without awakening until 5:00 a.m. to 6:00 a.m. He estimates getting 5 or fewer hours of sleep each night. He does not have a history of snoring or witnessed apneas. He does not describe symptoms of restless legs syndrome, daytime sleepiness, or fatigue. He functions well during the day. He has always received high recommendations at his job. He denies symptoms of depression or other psychologic disorders. His sleep pattern is the same on weekends and during vacations. He is concerned because his wife falls asleep quickly at 10:00 p.m. and sleeps soundly for 8 hours, while he remains awake during the night. His medical history is unremarkable and he is taking no prescription medications. Physical examination is unremarkable and laboratory studies obtained from his primary care physician are all normal. What would you recommend next?
    A. Order 2 weeks of sleep diaries and actigraphy as well as polysomnography
    B. Initiate treatment with zaleplon 5 mg at bedtime
    C. Initiate treatment with ramelteon
    D. Reassure him that his sleep pattern is normal and that no further work-up is necessary

186. Which of the following medications is most commonly associated with the development of REM sleep behavior disorder?
    A. Paroxetine
    B. Simvastatin
    C. Verapamil
    D. Zolpidem

187. Which of the following mechanisms related to pathophysiology of obesity hypoventilation syndrome is correct?
    A. Reduction in mechanical load on the chest wall and lungs associated with obesity
    B. Increased central ventilatory responses to hypoxemia and hypercapnia
    C. Increased upper airway resistance during sleep
    D. Increased sensitivity to the effects of leptin

188. A patient wishes to discuss surgical options for the treatment of obstructive sleep apnea (OSA). Which of the following statements is true related to surgical treatment of OSA?
    A. Uvulopalatopharyngoplasty (UPPP) has an overall success rate of 40% in a meta-analysis published in 1996
    B. UPPP can be expected to have a probability of successful treatment of OSA of approximately 85% to 90% based on a criteria of reduction in the apnea–hypopnea index (AHI) to less than 5 events per hour
    C. The probability of treatment success of UPPP can be accurately predicted by cephalometric radiographs
    D. Patients with primarily hypopharyngeal collapse identified by flexible laryngoscopy during a Muller maneuver have the highest probability of success from UPPP

189. Which of the following statements regarding the relationship between obstructive sleep apnea (OSA) and pulmonary hypertension is true?
    A. Most patients with OSA have significant pulmonary hypertension identified by echocardiography
    B. Patients who have OSA with severe oxygen desaturation are more likely to have elevations in pulmonary artery pressure than patients with OSA but without severe oxygen desaturation
    C. Bosentan is the preferred first-line agent for the treatment of pulmonary hypertension due to OSA
    D. All patients diagnosed with OSA should have an echocardiogram to identify pulmonary hypertension

190. Which of the following statements regarding the cardiovascular effects of obstructive sleep apnea (OSA) is true?
    A. OSA is an independent risk factor of the development of atrial fibrillation
    B. The presence of obesity, but not OSA, is associated with increased mortality from cardiovascular disease
    C. OSA is associated with a greater risk for ventricular dysrhythmias but not atrial dysrhythmias
    D. In patients with OSA, atrial fibrillation is almost always seen in the presence of heart failure

191. Which of the following statements about patients with obstructive sleep apnea (OSA) syndrome is true?
    A. Compared to patients without OSA, patients with OSA are more likely to succumb to sudden cardiac death between the hours of midnight and 6:00 a.m. than during other hours of the day
    B. Compared to patients without OSA, they are no more likely to succumb to sudden cardiac death between midnight and 6:00 a.m. than during other hours of the day
    C. In patients without OSA, a peak incidence of sudden death occurs between midnight and 6:00 a.m.
    D. There is no significant temporal pattern to the incidence of sudden cardiac death

192. Which of the following sleep disturbances is most commonly seen in patients with Alzheimer disease (AD)?
    A. Increase in number of REM periods, increased REM density, and a shortened initial REM latency
    B. Alteration in circadian rhythmicity with reversal of the usual day–night wake–sleep pattern
    C. REM sleep behavior disorder is commonly observed in the early stages of AD or preceding the diagnosis
    D. Normal sleep architecture on polysomnography

193. **In patients with seasonal affective disorder (SAD), which of the following regimens of light therapy is recommended?**
    A. 2,500 lux for 90 minutes in the late afternoon
    B. 2,500 lux for 30 minutes in the evening prior to bedtime
    C. 10,000 lux for 30 minutes in the morning after awakening
    D. 10,000 lux for 2 hours in the morning after awakening

194. **A 20-year-old college student seeks consultation for excessive daytime sleepiness. She is a junior college student at a large state university. She relates sleeping well while in elementary school or in high school when she received high grades and was able to engage in a variety of extracurricular activities. Over the last 2 years, however, she has trouble falling asleep at night as well as difficulty waking up to go to class in the morning. She has fallen asleep in class on several occasions. At one time, she slept through an examination scheduled at 9:00 a.m. and received a failing grade. On weeknights, she stays up until 2:00 a.m., at which time she falls asleep quickly. She cannot wake up early in the morning. She finds herself falling asleep frequently during her classes. On weekends, she sleeps until noon or 1:00 p.m. She does not feel rested during the day, but does not fall asleep involuntarily in the afternoons or evenings. She seems to have a burst of energy in the evening and does her school work during these hours. She has read about narcolepsy and believes that it may be her problem. She denies cataplexy, although she occasionally has experienced sleep paralysis upon arising in the morning. She does not describe hypnagogic hallucinations. Past medical history is complete. Her physical examination is normal. What would be the next diagnostic step for this patient?**
    A. Polysomnography and multiple sleep latency test
    B. Sleep diary for 2 weeks
    C. HLA profile looking for DQB1*0602 allele
    D. Cerebrospinal fluid hypocretin level

195. **Which of the following physiologic changes involving respiration occurs during stable NREM sleep compared to wakefulness?**
    A. Decrease in $PaCO_2$
    B. Relative increase in ventilation due to hyperventilation
    C. Relative decrease in ventilation due to bronchoconstriction
    D. Relative decrease in ventilation due to an increase in upper airway resistance

196. **Stimulus control therapy (SCT) is commonly used to treat insomnia. Which of the following statements best describes the principle underlying this technique?**
    A. SCT is based on the principle of operant conditioning, suggesting that wakefulness is indirectly rewarding and therefore maintained
    B. SCT is based on the principle of classical conditioning by pairing waking activities with the sleep environment, thereby making the sleep environment a discriminative cue for increased arousal

C. SCT is based on the principle that individuals with cognitive issues of control attempt to control their sleep and become alert by trying to sleep

D. SCT is based on the principle that underlying all insomnia is a weak homeostatic drive and that, by controlling bedtime, the drive can be increased

197. What is rebound insomnia?

A. Sleep that is worse than baseline following rapid time zone travel

B. Sleep that is worse than baseline occurring after a period of extended sleep (Sunday night insomnia)

C. Sleep that is worse than baseline following discontinuation of hypnotic medications

D. Return of poor sleep following a period of relatively good sleep

198. The specific difference between panic disorder and generalized anxiety disorder (GAD) is the presence of panic attacks. Which of the following statements regarding the sleep of individuals with panic disorder is true?

A. Panic attacks typically occur during wakefulness and are very unusual during sleep

B. Sleep panic attacks are distinguishable from nightmares or sleep terrors

C. In contrast to patients with GAD, panic disorder patients often sleep quite well because they do not experience panic attacks during sleep

D. Sleep phobia is unusual as a result of panic attacks

199. What is the most stable objective change seen in the sleep in individuals with schizophrenia?

A. Consistently shortened REM latency

B. REM sleep abnormalities that underly the hallucinations of schizophrenic patients

C. Changes in NREM sleep with deficits of N3 sleep or reduced delta wave activity

D. Robust rebound of N3 sleep following sleep deprivation

200. The reticular activating system (RAS) contains three main nuclei, pedunculopontine nucleus (PPN), the raphe nucleus (RN), and locus coeruleus (LC). All three of these nuclei are active during wakefulness. How do these nuclei respond during sleep?

A. All three continue to fire at a constant rate during NREM and REM sleep but less than during wakefulness

B. All three essentially cease to fire during both NREM and REM sleep

C. During REM sleep, the PPN is very active, while the LC and RN are almost silent

D. During REM sleep, the LC and RN are very active, while the PPN is almost silent

201. What effect would blocking the output of the tuberomammillary nucleus (TMN) have on behavior?

A. Increased alertness

B. Increased sleepiness

C. No significant effect on sleep

D. Increased motor activity but little effect on sleepiness or alertness

202. **Which of the following statements best characterizes recovery sleep following a period of total sleep deprivation?**
A. The majority of N3 sleep is recovered
B. The majority of REM sleep is recovered
C. The majority of N2 sleep is recovered
D. All sleep stages increase modestly but a clear deficit of all stages remains

203. **What is the specific mechanism of action of modafinil?**
A. Dopamine agonist
B. Adenosine antagonist
C. Histamine agonist
D. Unknown

204. **Individuals who smoke cigarettes often report that smoking has a calming effect. Which of the following is true of nicotine administration?**
A. Smoking can increase both snoring and obstructive sleep apnea
B. Transdermal nicotine delivery is associated with improved sleep
C. Sleep disturbance is associated with nicotine use but not during withdrawal
D. Smoking at bedtime decreases sleep latency

205. **What is the most predominant symptom of Kleine–Levin syndrome?**
A. Periodic hypersomnia
B. Periodic insomnia
C. Hypersexuality
D. Cataplexy

206. **Nocturia can develop in adults with obstructive sleep apnea (OSA). Which of the following is considered a factor in nocturia associated with OSA?**
A. Increase in urinary concentrating ability
B. Decreased excretion of atrial natriuretic peptide
C. Decreased intra-abdominal pressure
D. Awareness of urinary pressure during arousals

207. **A 54-year-old woman is seen for chronic insomnia dating back to her mid-20s. She reports sleep onset and maintenance insomnia with a perceived sleep-onset latency of 45 minutes, three to five awakenings during the night, and one or two episodes of nocturia. She admits to persistent mental activation at sleep onset. There is a relevant past medical history of depression. She had been prescribed citalopram years ago; her primary care physician recently suggested reinitiation of the therapy. She had reinitiated the therapy but felt it did not improve her sleep and discontinued the medication. The patient is unaware if she snores during sleep but denied awakenings with a gasping sensation. The patient admits to nocturnal perspiration but denied morning headaches. She started her menopause 2 years ago and has gained 24 lb since that time. Her vital**

signs are normal except for a body mass index (BMI) of 29. Upper oral airway examination reveals a Mallampati class 4 airway. Tonsils are not visible. She has a broad tongue. The remaining physical examination is normal.

What is the most desirable clinical action at this time?

A. Provide a prescription for zolpidem 10 mg to be taken at bedtime with a follow-up visit in 1 month

B. Refer the patient for cognitive behavioral therapy for insomnia (CBT-I)

C. Refer the patient for psychiatric evaluation

D. Provide a prescription for ramelteon 8 mg to be taken at bedtime and request a diagnostic polysomnography

208. You see a 23-year-old single male who is referred for consultation due to difficulty initiating sleep and excessive sleepiness. He has experienced recurrent difficulties with sleep-onset insomnia since age 15. He indicates that his current difficulties started 6 months ago, following his college graduation and start of his first job as a research assistant. He reports a bedtime of 10:00 p.m. with an estimated sleep-onset latency of 3 hours. Once asleep, he reports no awakenings but has extreme difficulty arising at 5:30 a.m. He has an alarm clock at the bedside and three alarms programmed on his cellular phone. Yet he requires a call from his girlfriend to make sure he gets out of bed on time. He suffered from panic attacks in his teens and was managed on alprazolam 0.25 mg. He denied symptoms of depression. His affect was somewhat anxious. He described his neighborhood as quite noisy before 10:00 p.m. His room is not dark and the light from the street reflects through his bedroom window. His girlfriend has noted snoring but is not concerned about his breathing during sleep. However, she has asked him to pursue consultation because he experiences significant sleepiness when driving to work in the morning. His score on the Epworth Sleepiness Scale is 7. The patient has no clinical evidence of cataplexy or hypnagogic hallucinations but has experienced sleep paralysis on awakening. His physical examination is unremarkable.

On the basis of the above information, what is the most desirable clinical action at this time?

A. Review sleep hygiene, prescribe eszopiclone 3 mg at bedtime, and have the patient return for follow-up in 1 month

B. Initiate citalopram 10 mg daily and recommend counseling to help minimize anxiety associated with the new job

C. Review stimulus control, prescribe zaleplon 20 mg at bedtime, and have the patient return in 1 month

D. Order diagnostic polysomnography followed by a multiple sleep latency test to evaluate the patient's sleep-related symptoms

209. You recently ordered a multiple sleep latency test (MSLT) and after reviewing the tracing determine that the report does not match your estimated sleep-onset latencies. In reviewing the discrepancy in the scoring of the test, you decide to give instructions to the sleep laboratory

technologist on how to rescore the test. What is the most appropriate instruction when scoring sleep-onset latency on an MSLT?

A. Score from the beginning of the test to the first minute of any stage of sleep

B. Score from the beginning of the test to the first epoch of N1 sleep that is followed by an additional two consecutive epochs of N1 sleep

C. Score from the beginning of the test to the first epoch containing 15 seconds of any stage of sleep

D. Score from the first epoch of sleep to the first epoch of REM sleep

210. A 48-year-old man presents with a history of loud, disruptive snoring and witnessed apneas during sleep. His score on the Epworth Sleepiness Scale is 9. Overnight ambulatory oximetry revealed an oxygen desaturation index of 30 per hour with an average oxygen saturation of 91% and a lowest oxygen saturation of 75%. The patient is interested in discussing potential therapeutic interventions to address a presumed diagnosis of obstructive sleep apnea (OSA). Of the following options, which one would be the best clinical advice at this time?

A. Conservative therapy with weight loss and good sleep hygiene practices with follow-up clinic visit in 3 months

B. Split-night polysomnography followed by implementation of bi-level positive airway pressure therapy

C. Split-night polysomnography followed by implementation of continuous positive airway pressure therapy

D. Follow up with otolaryngology referral

211. An 18-year-old woman is referred for symptoms of excessive sleepiness. She has been followed by a psychiatrist for treatment of auditory hallucinations, which have been partially controlled with quetiapine 50 mg at bedtime. The clinical assessment reveals that the patient has no symptoms consistent with a psychiatric disorder. Auditory hallucinations are only associated with sleep onset. She initially noted the symptoms of excessive sleepiness during her first year in high school. She denied symptoms consistent with sleep paralysis or cataplexy. She follows a regular sleep schedule and there is no evidence of insufficient sleep. There is no history of recreational drug use. She has a roommate who has not been aware of snoring. The patient's medical history and physical examination are otherwise noncontributory. Which of the following is the most desirable course of action at this time?

A. Increase the dose of quetiapine and ask the patient to keep a sleep diary for 1 month to further characterize her sleep schedule

B. Stop quetiapine, initiate lorazepam 0.5 mg at bedtime, and order a diagnostic polysomnography

C. Continue quetiapine at bedtime and initiate modafinil 200 mg every morning

D. Stop quetiapine, keep the patient medication free for 2 weeks, and then have the patient complete an overnight diagnostic polysomnography followed by a multiple sleep latency test (MSLT) the following day

212. A 49-year-old man is seen in consultation for a second opinion. He has a previous diagnosis of obstructive sleep apnea. The diagnosis was established 6 weeks ago and an apnea–hypopnea index of 48 is documented on the polysomnographic report. The patient completed continuous positive airway pressure (CPAP) titration under a split-night protocol and was prescribed CPAP at 11 cm H_2O. He reports nightly use and his score on the Epworth Sleepiness Scale (ESS) at the time of your consultation is 8. The patient reports no difficulties with CPAP and requests you to write a letter to his flight surgeon releasing him to return to work as a commercial pilot.

   On the basis of the available information, what is the best course of action to take at this time?
   A. Allow him to return to work
   B. Prescribe modafinil 200 mg daily and release him to return to work
   C. Advise the patient that the Federal Aviation Administration (FAA) requires him to have a score of 5 on the ESS
   D. Advise the patient that the FAA requires him to pass a maintenance of wakefulness test (MWT)

213. You are asked to see in consultation a 32-year-old truck driver. He is referred by his primary care physician because of treatment-resistant hypertension. He lives alone and he denies any sleep-related symptoms. His score on the Epworth Sleepiness Scale (ESS) is 4. When you question the patient about his sleep schedule practices, he replies that he sleeps "here and there." You are unable to fully characterize his sleep schedule practices. On the basis of the available information, what is the best recommendation at this time?
   A. Five days of actigraphy to fully characterize the patient's sleep schedules
   B. Two weeks of sleep logs to characterize the patient's sleep–wake schedule
   C. Schedule diagnostic polysomnography
   D. Recommend implementation of improved sleep hygiene practices

214. You are called by a colleague who has been treating a 55-year-old woman for the past 6 months. The patient has significant insomnia in the context of a history of depression and has developed tolerance to sleep medications that have been previously prescribed. Your colleague has been prescribing alprazolam 1.5 mg at bedtime with only partial resolution of the patient's difficulty initiating sleep. What is your advice to your colleague?
   A. Request sleep medicine consultation
   B. Switch from alprazolam to clonazepam 1.0 mg
   C. Add eszopiclone 2 mg at bedtime
   D. Adjust alprazolam to 2.0 mg at bedtime

215. You are reviewing the results of a diagnostic polysomnography completed on a 36-year-old woman. The sleep laboratory data revealed a sleep efficiency of 88%. Time-in-bed period was 8 hours. Sleep-onset latency was 15 minutes. REM latency was 70 minutes. Sleep architecture and sleep continuity were preserved. The apnea–hypopnea index was 4 per hour. Laboratory technicians noted mild snoring. Oxygen saturation was stable

at levels above 90%. You review the postsleep questionnaire, which reflects the patient's estimates of her sleep in the laboratory. She estimated taking 1 hour to fall asleep and thought she slept 3 hours. What is your diagnosis based on the available information?

A. Insomnia due to mental disorder
B. Paradoxical insomnia
C. Behavioral insomnia of adulthood
D. Idiopathic insomnia

216. What is the pathognomonic symptom of narcolepsy?
    A. Hypnagogic hallucinations
    B. Cataplexy
    C. Sleep paralysis
    D. Excessive daytime sleepiness

217. A 26-year-old man presents with symptoms of excessive sleepiness. He describes sleep paralysis on awakening but no hypnagogic hallucinations or cataplexy. The patient's reported sleep schedule during the week is bedtime at midnight and arising time at 5:30 a.m. On weekends, bedtime is delayed to 2:00 a.m. and arising time is 7:00 a.m. What is your recommendation to the patient?
    A. Start modafinil 200 mg each morning
    B. Improve sleep schedule practices by regularizing and increasing time in bed; ask the patient to keep a sleep log and return for follow-up in 1 month
    C. Schedule overnight diagnostic polysomnography followed by a multiple sleep latency test
    D. Determine cerebrospinal fluid (CSF) hypocretin-1 levels

218. You are asked to see a 56-year-old woman with a previous diagnosis of generalized anxiety disorder (GAD). Her psychiatrist has been treating her with paroxetine 40 mg daily and clonazepam 1 mg four times a day. Her symptoms of GAD have remained under good control for a number of years. She was referred for assessment of excessive daytime sleepiness. She reports increasing levels of sleepiness across the day with significant sleepiness when driving in the evening. The assessment does not reveal clinical evidence of other relevant sleep-related conditions. What is your best advice based on the available information?
    A. Prescribe modafinil 200 mg daily
    B. Prescribe methylphenidate 5 mg
    C. Taper clonazepam and determine if it is possible to discontinue the benzodiazepine
    D. Replace clonazepam with lorazepam 0.5 mg four times a day

219. You see a 39-year-old female with a complaint of excessive sleepiness. Polysomnographic assessment revealed reduced sleep efficiency and increased frequency of awakenings. There was no evidence of sleep-related breathing disorder, restless legs, or periodic limb movements. Multiple sleep latency test (MSLT) revealed an average sleep-onset latency of 9 minutes and one sleep-onset REM period. The patient reported

occasional use of alcoholic beverages but has had no consumption in the last month. The patient has recently displayed poor work attendance and spends the entire day in bed. She has manifested lack of interest as well as social withdrawal. Her most recent blood work revealed a marginal elevation in her cholesterol levels. What is the most likely diagnosis?

- A. Hypersomnia not due to substance or known physiologic condition
- B. Physiologic hypersomnia
- C. Hypersomnia due to medical condition
- D. Narcolepsy due to medical condition

220. **Which of the following statements most accurately describes the currently available subjective sleepiness scales?**
- A. The Stanford Sleepiness Scale represents an adequate scale for the clinical assessment of excessive sleepiness
- B. A score of 6 on the Epworth Sleepiness Scale (ESS) is indicative of excessive sleepiness
- C. The Sleep–Wake Activity Inventory (SWAI) – EDS Scale is most useful in the assessment of circadian rhythm disorders
- D. Both the ESS and the SWAI were validated against the multiple sleep latency test (MSLT)

221. **Of the following options, which one is considered an adequate tool in the assessment of circadian rhythm disorders?**
- A. Sleep–Wake Activity Inventory (SWAI) – EDS Scale
- B. Stanford Sleepiness Scale
- C. The dim-light melatonin onset
- D. Epworth Sleepiness Scale

222. **Which of the following events indicates tonic REM sleep?**
- A. Muscle atonia
- B. Autonomic irregularities
- C. Rapid eye movements
- D. Ponto-geniculate-occipital (PGO) waves

223. **Which of the following does not represent characteristics of ponto-geniculate-occipital (PGO) waves?**
- A. They herald the onset of REM sleep
- B. They are generated in the rostral pontine reticular formation near the cerebellum
- C. They are present during tonic REM sleep
- D. They activate gamma aminobutyric acid (GABA)ergic neurons that serve to inhibit cortical activity

224. **Which of the following is considered a manifestation of the homeostatic response to sleep deprivation?**
- A. Decreased auditory awakening thresholds
- B. Increased N3 sleep
- C. Increased sleep-onset latency
- D. Decreased total sleep time

225. **What is the REM latency that reflects a sleep-onset REM period (SOREMP) on a multiple sleep latency test?**
    A. REM latency of 10 minutes
    B. REM latency of 20 minutes
    C. REM latency of 30 minutes
    D. REM latency of 50 minutes

226. **You have completed an overnight REM sleep deprivation study on a group of eight alert, healthy subjects. Which one of the statements best reflects your expected result?**
    A. Decreased sleep-onset latencies on the multiple sleep latency test (MSLT)
    B. Unchanged sleep-onset latencies on the MSLT
    C. Multiple sleep-onset REM periods on the MSLT
    D. At least one subject will be expected to experience psychotic symptoms as a result of REM deprivation

227. **What is the definition of pharmacologic tolerance?**
    A. Progressive increases in the doses of a medication are required to achieve the desired effect
    B. Physiologic changes that are characterized by withdrawal symptoms
    C. Maladaptive pattern of drug use
    D. Rebound phenomena with worsening of the underlying symptoms

228. **Which one of the following medications is not considered a predisposing/precipitating factor in the manifestation of REM sleep behavior disorder?**
    A. Venlafaxine
    B. Sertraline
    C. Paroxetine
    D. Bupropion

229. **Which one of the following medications has the highest risk of causing excessive daytime sedation?**
    A. Zolpidem
    B. Triazolam
    C. Eszopiclone
    D. Flurazepam

230. **Which one of the following characteristics reflects polysomnographic evidence of insomnia?**
    A. Sleep-onset latency – 30 minutes
    B. Sleep efficiency – 95%
    C. Number of awakenings – 10/hour
    D. Stage 1 NREM sleep percent – <30%

231. **Which one of the following hypnotic medications is more likely to shorten sleep-onset latency while being the least likely to cause residual sedation?**
    A. Zolpidem 10 mg at bedtime
    B. Eszopiclone 1 mg at bedtime
    C. Eszopiclone 3 mg at bedtime
    D. Zaleplon 20 mg at bedtime

232. **You are asked to give an opinion about the effectiveness of the different therapeutic modalities in the management of obstructive sleep apnea (OSA). Among the following statements, which is the most credible?**
    A. Continuous positive airway pressure (CPAP) is 100% effective in the treatment of OSA
    B. Uvulopalatopharyngoplasty (UPPP) reduces the apnea–hypopnea index (AHI), on average, by 80%
    C. A recent prospective, randomized study of the Pillar procedure documented this treatment to be superior to placebo with 70% of subjects achieving a reduction in the AHI of >50% versus 20% in the placebo group
    D. A contraindication for oral appliance therapy is a history of temporo-mandibular joint (TMJ) disease

233. **You have a 48-year-old man at the office for a 3-month follow-up visit. You had prescribed continuous positive airway pressure (CPAP) at 10 cm H_2O when you last saw him for treatment of severe obstructive sleep apnea (OSA) (apnea–hypopnea index [AHI] = 42 per hour). You are seeing him for the first time since the initiation of therapy. Of the following parameters, which one indicates the single least critical parameter in evaluating his CPAP adherence?**
    A. Average time used per day during the total period
    B. Percent of days used for the period being evaluated
    C. Average number of CPAP sessions per use days
    D. Average use/night on nights with CPAP utilization

234. **You have a 55-year-old woman at the office for a 3-month follow-up visit. You had adjusted her continuous positive airway pressure (CPAP) setting from 8 to 7 cm H_2O when you last saw her because of complaints of persistent leaks. The patient reports improved tolerance to therapy but admits to difficulty maintaining sleep with three nocturnal awakenings during the night. She acknowledges that she does not like to use the humidifier because it involves too much extra effort. She rates herself with a score of 12 on the Epworth Sleepiness Scale. The print out from the CPAP unit reflects CPAP use on 20% of the nights over the last 3 months. Nightly use of CPAP (on nights that CPAP was used) averaged 2 hours 6 minutes. The unit's estimated apnea–hypopnea index (AHI) is 5 per hour. The patient reports awareness of dry mouth upon awakening. You review with the patient a number of recommendations you would like her to implement. Which of the following indicates the best desirable recommendation based on the available information?**
    A. Encourage the use of the CPAP humidifier
    B. Change to bi-level positive airway pressure (BPAP)
    C. Prescribe eszopiclone 2 mg at bedtime
    D. Prescribe modafinil 100 mg daily

235. **You evaluate a 58-year-old man who sees you in consultation for a second opinion. He was diagnosed with obstructive sleep apnea (OSA) 6 months ago; continuous positive airway pressure (CPAP) was prescribed at 13 cm H_2O, and the patient reports a good experience with therapy. The print**

out from the unit confirms therapeutic response and adequate use. The patient perceives improved quality of sleep but has complained of persistent sleepiness. His treating physician ordered a multiple sleep latency test (MSLT). The patient brings the report for your review.

	Trial 1	Trial 2	Trial 3	Trial 4	Trial 5	
Start Time	8:00	10:00	12:00	14:00	16:00	
Onset to Sleep (min)	4.0	6.5	7.0	2.0	8.0	Average = 6.5
Onset to REM Sleep (min)[A]	32.0	—	—	34.0	—	2 SOREMPs
End of Nap	8:40	10:40	12:40	14:40	16:40	
Recall Sleep?	Yes	No	No	Yes	No	
Pt latency estimate	5	—	—	5	—	

SOREMP, sleep-onset REM period.

The available information leads you to conclude that the patient should initiate modafinil 100 mg daily. Your written review of the MSLT report lists the following observations.

Which of these is correct?

A. The report suggests that the MSLT was not completed according to American Academy of Sleep Medicine (AASM) criteria

B. The interpretation correctly indicates the presence of polysomnographic evidence of narcolepsy

C. The correct average sleep-onset latency is 4.5 minutes

D. The patient's perception of sleep is critical to the interpretation of the test

236. A patient being treated for insomnia associated with major depressive disorder has been tried on a variety of sedative-hypnotic and antidepressant medications. Which is likely to suppress REM sleep the most?

A. Barbiturate pentobarbital

B. Benzodiazepine temazepam

C. Benzodiazepine receptor agonist zaleplon

D. Atypical antidepressant buspirone

237. Polysomnography is performed on a 26-year-old, otherwise healthy, man complaining of snoring and nocturnal gastroesophageal reflux. His body mass index is 21 and baseline oxygen saturations are above 96%. The patient has a mixture of respiratory effort–associated arousals associated with snoring and several episodes in which central sleep apnea episodes occur. Arterial blood gases would most likely reveal that the patient has which of the following acid–base abnormalities?

A. Hypocapnic

B. Eucapnic

C. Hypercapnia

D. Hypoxemia

238. A 6-ft-tall, 65-year-old man with a body mass index of 26 has a 10-year history of insomnia. He practices good sleep hygiene and does not snore or suffer from excessive sleepiness. His wife confirms this report. Pulmonary function testing reveals an FEV_1/FVC ratio of 60% and an FEV_1 that is 50% of the predicted value. Although he has chronic nocturnal cough during the early part of the sleep period, his main insomnia complaint is that he awakens at 1:30 a.m. gasping for breath. What is the most likely cause of his insomnia?

A. Severe, undiagnosed obstructive sleep apnea

B. Psychogenic choking

C. Major depressive disorder

D. Hyperinflation and ventilation–perfusion mismatching

239. A 72-in-tall, 230-lb, 55-year-old woman presents with a complaint of sleep maintenance insomnia. The problem began approximately 2 years ago and seems to be getting progressively worse. She also notes increasing nocturia and dreaming. Her physician recommended hormone replacement therapy about 3 years ago but she opted to not fill the prescription because her hot flashes were not severe and she had health-related concerns. Her blood pressure is slightly elevated for which she takes diuretics. She is a trial lawyer and is mainly distressed because her memory is not as sharp as it used to be and she can no longer work late nights productively, notwithstanding her difficulty sleeping. What is the most likely cause of her insomnia?

A. Postmenopausal-related obstructive sleep apnea

B. Bipolar disorder

C. Early Alzheimer disease

D. Periodic limb movement disorder

240. A well-dressed, 24-year-old, 5 ft 7 in, 155-lb, married woman presents at the sleep center with extreme daytime sleepiness that began suddenly several weeks before. She retires for sleep at 10:30 p.m. and arises at 6:30 a.m. on weekdays and maintains the same schedule on weekends. Overall, she is very health conscious, jazzercises regularly, does yoga, and maintains very good nutrition. She has no prior history of sleepiness, does not snore, and reports sleeping well. There is no family history of narcolepsy, obstructive sleep apnea, or other disorders of excessive somnolence. Beck Depression Inventory score is 6 and Epworth Sleepiness Scale score is 21. She was scheduled for an overnight polysomnography and a multiple sleep latency test, but called a week before the sleep study to cancel the tests, explaining that she is no longer sleepy and the reason why she was sleepy is now apparent. Which of the following was the reason for her complaint?

A. Kleine–Levin Syndrome

B. Recurrent idiopathic torpor

C. Cocaine withdrawal

D. Pregnancy

241. **Although the hypnotoxin model of sleep regulation predicts that sleepiness is a function of the length of prior wakefulness, it is well known that most individuals arising in the morning do not get progressively sleepier as the day progresses and that peak alertness is reached in the mid- to late evening. What is the best explanation for this?**
    A. Homeostatic mechanism periodically decreases because of metabolic factors and overall downregulation
    B. Liver enzymes clear circulating hypnotoxins, producing renewed receptor sensitivity
    C. Circadian sleep–wake pacemaker increases its output until melatonin shuts it down
    D. Circadian variation in cortisol levels across the day to offset increasing sleep drive

242. **According to the activation-synthesis hypothesis of dream formation, which of the following statements is correct?**
    A. Dreams are the result of specifically activated subcortical areas that release preprogrammed cortical areas to facilitate memory encoding of recently learned information
    B. Dreams are activated from encapsulated memories that are released by cerebellar inhibition
    C. Dreams are archetypal manifestations of genetic and racial synthesized memories that exist in all humans
    D. Dreams are formed when the cortex makes its best attempt to make sense out of the random activity arising from the brainstem

243. **A 42-year-old woman with a chief complaint of insomnia has an overnight polysomnography for suspected obstructive sleep apnea. She, however, has no evidence of sleep-disordered breathing or upper airway resistance syndrome. She complains of both difficulty initiating and maintaining sleep. According to the patient, her sleep is not related to pain but there is a past history of depression. Abnormalities in both sleep micro- and macroarchitecture are noted. Which abnormality would likely have been observed?**
    A. REM sleep latency of 45 minutes
    B. Slow-wave sleep percentage that is above normal for her age
    C. Decreased beta activity
    D. Low REM density

244. **A 22-year-old, 5 ft 5 in, 170-lb, woman with suspected narcolepsy has an overnight polysomnography followed the next day by a multiple sleep latency test (MSLT). The patient reports symptoms of sleepiness, hypnagogic hallucinations, sleep paralysis, teeth grinding, snoring, and nightmares. The overnight polysomnography begins at 10:30 p.m. and ends at 6:00 a.m. with a sleep efficiency of 80%, sleep latency of 3 minutes, REM sleep percentage of 18%, REM sleep latency of 38 minutes, and no slow-wave sleep. The apnea–hypopnea index is 2.1 and respiratory disturbance index (RDI) is only 4.5 events per hour of sleep. Bruxism is noted during the first NREM episode but does not reoccur. The first MSLT nap opportunity begins at 8:15 a.m., has a sleep onset on epoch 9,**

and REM sleep occurs on epochs 15 through 25. The second nap opportunity begins at 10:00 a.m., has a sleep onset on epoch 12, and REM sleep does not occur. The third nap opportunity reveals sleep onset at epoch 3 but no REM sleep is noted. Finally, in the fourth nap opportunity, the patient falls asleep on epoch 8 but there is no REM sleep during the following 15 minutes. What conclusions would you reach on the basis of these findings?

A. The tests confirm that the patient has narcolepsy
B. The tests confirm that the patient does not have narcolepsy
C. The tests are inconclusive because MSLT was improperly conducted
D. The tests are inconclusive because results were equivocal

245. A 31-year-old man is referred to the sleep clinic after injuring himself during sleep. He lives and sleeps alone and, several times in the past, has awakened to find himself out of his bed. He has a history of asthma, depression, anxiety, and kidney stones. He takes a multivitamin, fish oil pills, a baby aspirin, and fluoxetine daily. Occasionally, he takes diazepam to help him sleep. His paternal uncle died of cystic fibrosis and his father has chronic obstructive pulmonary disease resulting from a long history of cigarette smoking. The rest of the family history is unremarkable. The episode that led to his referral was his arising from bed thinking there was a rat in his bedroom, chasing it to the corner and kicking it with his foot. In the dream, the rat was biting him. In actuality, he was kicking the fins of a baseboard heater and developed self-inflicted severe injury in the process. Upon awakening and noting that he was bleeding profusely, he rushed to the fire station across the street, arriving just before losing consciousness from loss of blood. What is the most likely explanation for this episode?

A. Sleepwalking provoked by his use of diazepam as a sedative-hypnotic agent
B. A fugue exacerbated by his anxiety disorder
C. REM sleep behavior disorder incited by his antidepressant agent
D. A sleep-related dissociative disorder prodromal for a recurrence of a major depressive episode

246. A 48-year-old man with a history of sleep apnea and treated with positive airway pressure is scheduled for a re-titration because of symptom recurrence and 20 lb weight gain. During polysomnography, the activity in Figure 14 is observed early in the night but did not recur. What would be the best therapeutic recommendation in this case?

A. Ignore the electroencephalographic activity because it is of no clinical significance
B. Begin antiepileptic treatment in response to the abnormal electroencephalography
C. Begin supplemental oxygen to treat his hypoxic seizures
D. Refer to neurology and include this sample of spike and wave with the clinical report

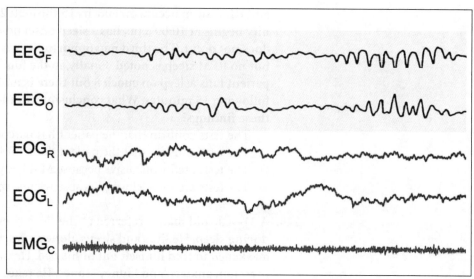

Figure 14.

247. **Which of the following statements accurately describes changes occurring in REM sleep during some part of the lifespan?**
    A. REM sleep (active sleep) amounts to 50% of total sleep time at birth and decrease to 30% by the end of the first year
    B. REM sleep remains stable at 20% to 25% of total sleep time during adulthood and then rapidly declines to less than 15% after 65 years of age
    C. REM sleep is significantly higher in men than in women throughout the lifespan
    D. At birth, sleep is marked by REM sleep (active sleep) occurring first and then followed by NREM (quiet sleep), but it reverts to the adult pattern at 3 years of age

248. **A 22-year-old soldier is diagnosed with posttraumatic stress disorder (PTSD), alcohol abuse, insomnia, and periodic limb movement disorder. Aside from these conditions, he appears to be in reasonably good health. He is treated with eye movement desensitization and reprocessing therapy in combination with administration of a selective serotonin reuptake inhibitor (SSRI), a dopamine agonist for his leg movements, and a benzodiazepine receptor agonist (BZRA) for insomnia. The patient is brought to the emergency room with multiple lacerations and a shoulder fracture after having dove off the end of the bed and through his bedroom window. The patient likely has which of the following?**
    A. REM sleep behavior disorder provoked by the SSRI and PTSD
    B. A severe case of sleepwalking induced by the BZRA
    C. Nocturnal fugue provoked by the dopamine agonist
    D. Seizure disorder

249. **Cognitive behavioral therapy for insomnia is most likely to include which of the following?**
    A. Universal sleep hygiene, stimulus control therapy, and sleep restriction therapy

B. Universal sleep hygiene, progressive relaxation therapy, eye movement desensitization, and reprocessing therapy

C. Universal sleep hygiene, sleep restriction therapy, and transactional therapy

D. Universal sleep hygiene, guided imagery, and systematic desensitization

250. **An overnight polysomnogram is recorded with three electroencephalographic derivations as follows:**

Channel 1: FZ-F3; high-pass filter set to 0.3 Hz; low-pass filter set to 35 Hz

Channel 2: C3-A2; high-pass filter set to 1.0 Hz; low-pass filter set to 35 Hz

Channel 3: OZ-CZ; high-pass filter set to 0.3 Hz; low-pass filter set to 35 Hz

Which of the channels is/are set up for proper recording according to the *American Academy of Sleep Medicine (AASM) Standardized Manual*?

A. Channel 1

B. Channel 2

C. Channel 3

D. Channels 1 and 2

251. **A 37-year-old, mildly obese, single woman with a history of peptic ulcer disease, panic attacks, and arthritis presents with chronic insomnia. She is a night shift worker with a usual weekday bedtime of 9:00 a.m. and arising time of 5:00 p.m. Sleep schedule during weekends is similar to that during weekdays, with a maximum shift in bed, arising, and total time in bed of less than 1 hour. Even though she keeps her sleep schedule shifted, carefully maintains a regular exercise schedule, and eats meals at the same time every day, she becomes very sleepy between 3:00 a.m. and 5:00 a.m. She drinks one to two 8-oz cups of coffee at midnight, which helps her maintain wakefulness. After work, she drives home, eats a light meal, watches television for an hour, and goes to bed. She sleeps soundly for 3 to 4 hours; however, at around 12:30 p.m. she awakens, uses the bathroom, but then has difficulty going back to sleep. She sleeps on-and-off fitfully for the next 3 to 4 hours. She awakens somewhat refreshed but is distressed by her sleep maintenance problems. What best explains why the patient awakens between noon and 3:00 p.m. and is unable to fall back to consolidated sleep?**

A. Homeostatic drive to sleep is shifted because of eating in the morning and exposure to bright light

B. Increasing circadian alerting signal combined with the 3-hour depletion of sleep debt interferes with sleep maintenance

C. Environmental factors of light, heat, and noise interfere with sleep

D. Cortisol release is shifted to occur at about noon by the patient's previous day's sleep–wake schedule

252. **Which of the following provokes nightmares?**

A. Beta adrenergic blockers and therapy with alpha adrenergics (agonist or blockers)

B. Amphetamine withdrawal and therapy with traditional neuroleptics

C. Anticholinergic drugs and therapy with adenosine antagonists

D. Serotonin autoreceptor agonists and therapy with histamine agonists

253. Which of the following describes slow-wave sleep?
A. Controlled by secretion of growth hormone
B. The most important type of sleep which is why it occurs early in the night, is very difficult to deprive, and is directly responsible for circadian regulation
C. Shaped by thalamic gamma aminobutyric acid (GABA)ergic neurons in the reticular nucleus that surround the specific and nonspecific thalamocortical relay nuclei that pace the activity projected to the cortex
D. The biologic substrate of sleepwalking, sleep terrors, and rhythmic movement disorder

254. As a result of the 2005 National Institutes of Health State-of-Science conference on insomnia, which of the following statements is correct?
A. Pharmacotherapy is recommended only for short-term treatment
B. It was recommended that insomnia be considered a symptom and that treatment should be directed exclusively at the underlying etiology
C. Behavioral treatments should not be used except when other approaches have failed
D. It was recommended to consider insomnia in terms of primary and co-morbid rather than primary and secondary because the latter may lead to undertreatment

255. A 44-year-old commercial truck driver with diabetes and hypertension undergoes polysomnography and is diagnosed with obstructive sleep apnea. He is prescribed continuous positive airway pressure (CPAP). He denies being sleepy and wants to continue his occupation. However, the company he works for wants a medical letter indicating that he is "fit for duty." During his 30- to 90-day follow-up appointment, what types of evaluation would you conduct?
A. An overnight polysomnography followed by a multiple sleep latency test
B. An Epworth Sleepiness Scale and a psychomotor vigilance test
C. A CPAP utilization download and a maintenance of wakefulness test
D. A complete physical examination, hematology, blood chemistries, and a situational immobilization test

256. The activation-synthesis hypothesis attempts to explain dreaming in terms of which of the following?
A. Neuronal activation of sensory systems that allow synthesis of prototypical archetype representations from our unconscious
B. Release of underlying drive states that form images to express forbidden wishes and desires
C. Stimulation of organ systems that transmit impulses to the brain that interprets them in terms of basic physical needs
D. Impulses arising from the pons and producing traffic in ponto-geniculate-occipital (PGO) cortex circuits that are spun into a story by the cortex

257. Which of the following best describes the ventrolateral preoptic nucleus (VLPO)?
A. A group of hypothalamic neurons mainly active during REM sleep
B. Stimulates the locus coeruleus and raphe nuclei by releasing galanin and gamma aminobutyric acid (GABA)

C. Inhibited by noradrenaline and acetylcholine

D. Inactivated by prostaglandin D2

258. **Which of the following statements is true concerning the *American Academy of Sleep Medicine (AASM) Standardized Manual*'s recommendations for polysomnographic recordings?**
    A. Electroencephalography minimal sampling rate is the same as the minimum recommended for electrooculography (EOG) recording
    B. Electroencephalography-recommended sampling rate is defined by the speed of standard digital multiplexers
    C. One sample per second on respiratory channels meets minimum sampling requirements
    D. Sampling rates are based on Weiner's principle that you must sample at eight times the highest resolvable frequency

259. **A young adult healthy man who has no sleep disorders is kept in bed for several days in a constant, dimly lit environment. He is provided snacks approximately every hour. Core body temperature, which is monitored continuously, would most likely show which of the following patterns?**
    A. Temperature fluctuations revealing a circadian rhythm that is very close to 24 hours
    B. Temperature fluctuations revealing a quickly accelerating phase delay with a period close to 27 hours
    C. Rapid disentrainment of the temperature and sleep–wake rhythms
    D. Flattening of the peak-to-trough amplitude and a tendency toward an advancing sleep phase

260. **In humans, which of the following is the strongest zeitgeber?**
    A. Light
    B. Exercise
    C. Eating
    D. Work schedule

261. **A 22-year-old college student living in Oslo, Norway, routinely becomes dysthymic during the winter when it is very cold and dark most of the time. After she graduates, she moves to Irvine, California, where she has been accepted to the medical school. She notices that her usual depressed mode does not occur during her first year living in California. What is the most likely explanation?**
    A. California is so groovy
    B. Her diet improved as her lifestyle changed
    C. It was much warmer which made her happy
    D. The more southern latitude decreased the difference in light exposure during the winter compared to the summer

262. **Growth hormone release is strongly coupled to which of the following?**
    A. Onset of sleep
    B. Stage N2 sleep but will uncouple in response to jet lag
    C. Stage N3 sleep
    D. REM sleep

263. Cortisol release typically peaks at which of the following time period?
   A. Approximately 2 to 3 hours before bedtime when alertness is at its maximum
   B. Approximately 2 to 3 hours before awakening
   C. Around the time of awakening
   D. In the mid-afternoon in response to the circadian low

264. The polysomnographic sample illustrated in Figure 15 was recorded on a 43-year-old woman with a lifelong history of insomnia. The overall sleep macroarchitecture is within normal limits for sleep stage percentage, number of awakenings, latency to sleep, and sleep efficiency. The patient is diagnosed with paradoxical insomnia. The microarchitectural abnormality depicted in the figure is which of the following?
   A. Alpha-delta sleep pattern
   B. Mu rhythm
   C. Periorbital integrated potentials
   D. Cyclic alternating pattern

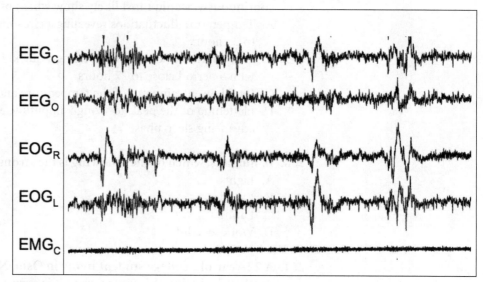

Figure 15.

265. A 22-year-old patient with a continuing history of substance abuse is brought into the emergency room by the police in a very agitated state. The police believed that he had overdosed on crack cocaine. Once in the emergency room, he becomes even more agitated and begins hallucinating. He is subsequently sedated and monitored for vital signs. He undergoes an unattended (but video-monitored) polysomnography. The activity shown in Figure 16 correlates with which sleep-related parasomnia?
   A. Rhythmic movement disorder
   B. Psychogenic choking
   C. Catathrenia
   D. Sleep bruxism

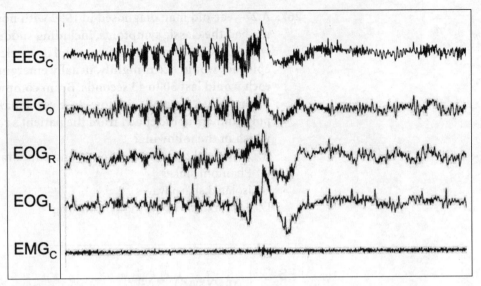

Figure 16.

266. A 66-year-old, thin (body mass index [BMI] <20) man with emphysema is evaluated polysomnographically and found not to have obstructive sleep apnea. However, prominent oxygen desaturation occurred during REM sleep. Early in the night, there is pronounced sleep continuity problems resulting from coughing. However, later in the night, the patient experiences episodes provoked by hyperinflation during which the following activity is noted on the polysomnogram. What best explains the activity depicted in the polysomnographic epoch shown in Figure 17?

A. Sweat artifact produced by respiratory effort
B. Hypersynchronous delta activity provoked by hyperthyroidism
C. Slow-wave sleep rebound from the earlier sleep loss due to coughing
D. Periodic lateralizing epileptiform discharges (PLEDs)

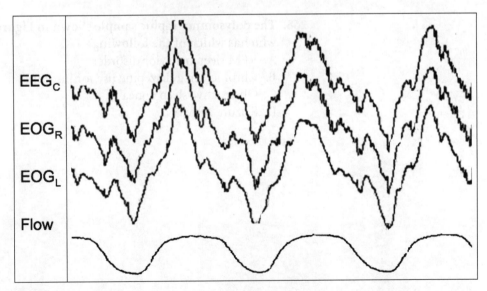

Figure 17.

267. A 27-year-old man diagnosed in 1992 with nocturnal paroxysmal dystonia had the classic symptoms, including sudden awakenings from sleep with choreoathetoid movements and dystonic posturing. Multiple episodes would occur nightly, usually emerging from stage N2 sleep, and each would last 30 to 45 seconds. Brain computed tomography is normal. The patient is treated with low-dose carbamazepine with good effect. The polysomnographic epoch from the patient's recording (see Fig. 18) shows which of the following?
    A. Abnormal flattening in frontal and temporal lobe activity
    B. Phantom spikes
    C. Isolated sharp waves
    D. Sawtooth theta during NREM sleep

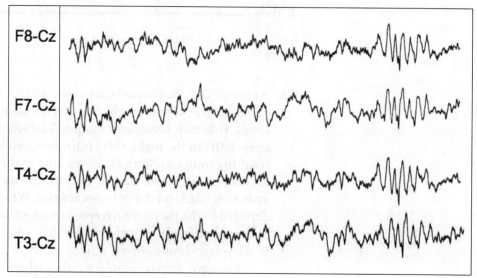

Figure 18.

268. The polysomnographic sample shown in Figure 19 is taken from a patient who has which of the following?
    A. REM sleep behavior disorder
    B. Chronic benzodiazepine use for insomnia
    C. Obstructive sleep apnea
    D. Seizure activity

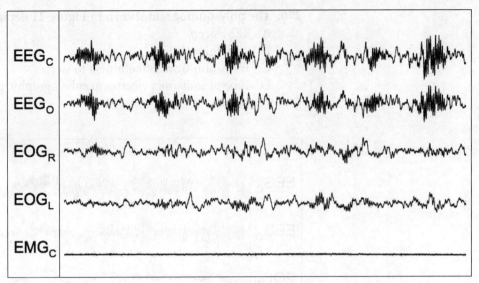

Figure 19.

269. The polysomnogram shown in Figure 20 is taken from a patient who most likely takes which of the following medications?
    A. Fluoxetine
    B. Benzodiazepines
    C. Beta encephalon agonist
    D. Clomipramine

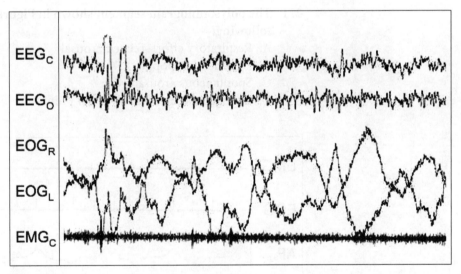

Figure 20.

270. **The polysomnogram shown in Figure 21 depicts which of the following?**
    A. REM sleep
    B. Wakefulness
    C. Transition from wakefulness to sleep
    D. Type of indistinct electroencephalographic pattern you see with sleep apnea

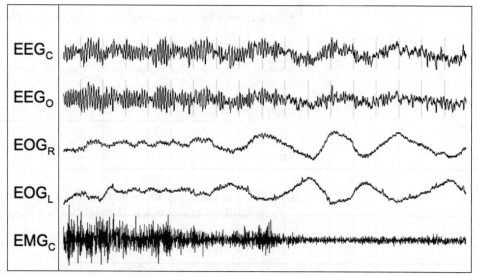

Figure 21.

271. **The polysomnogram segment shown in Figure 22 depicts which of the following?**
    A. Respiratory effort–related arousal
    B. Episode of hypopnea
    C. Spontaneous arousal
    D. Change in sleep respiratory set point

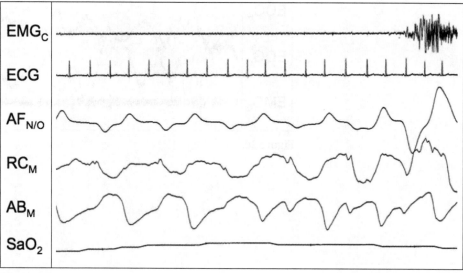

Figure 22.

272. **The polysomnographic sample shown in Figure 23 is representative of which of the following stages?**
    A. Stage of sleep that occurs 20% of the night
    B. Stage of sleep that occurs 30% of the night
    C. Stage of sleep that occurs 40% of the night
    D. Stage of sleep that occurs 50% of the night

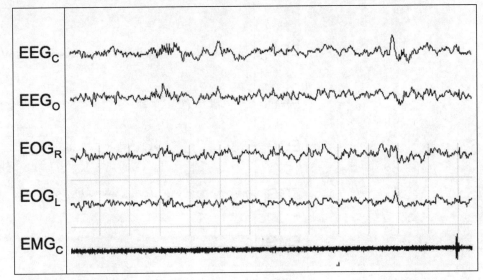

Figure 23.

273. **What best describes the polysomnographic epoch shown in Figure 24?**
    A. REM sleep
    B. Sleep onset
    C. Stage N1 sleep
    D. Arousal from REM sleep

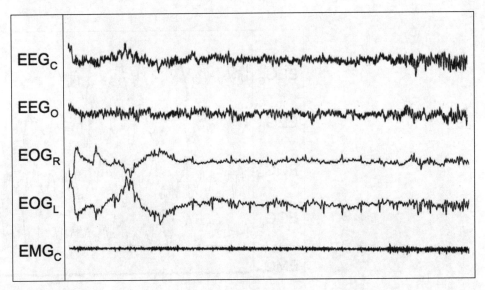

Figure 24.

274. **The polysomnographic epoch shown in Figure 25 depicts which of the following stage?**
    A. Stage N3
    B. Stage N2
    C. Stage N1
    D. Stage R

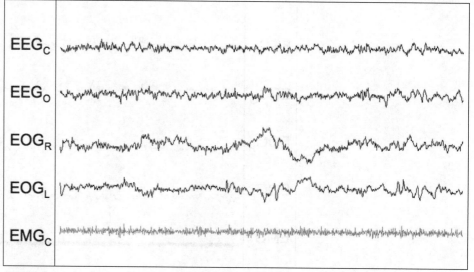

Figure 25.

275. **The polysomnographic epoch shown in Figure 26 depicts which of the following stage?**
    A. Stage N4
    B. Stage N3
    C. Stage N2
    D. Stage N1

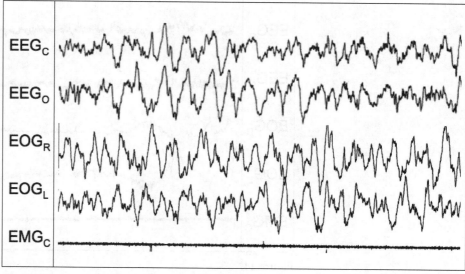

Figure 26.

276. **The polysomnographic segment illustrated in Figure 27 would be best described as showing which one of the following?**
    A. Epoch of stage N3 sleep
    B. Epoch of stage N2 sleep
    C. Arousal associated with a leg movement
    D. Movement artifact

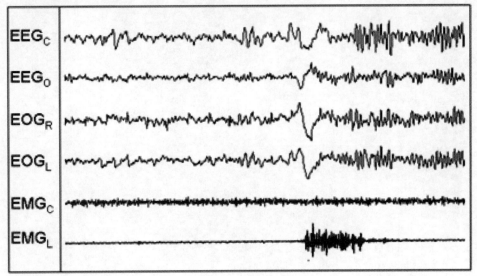

Figure 27.

277. **The respiratory event illustrated in Figure 28 is best described as which of the following?**
    A. Obstructive sleep apnea
    B. Obstructive sleep hypopnea
    C. Central apnea
    D. Mixed apnea

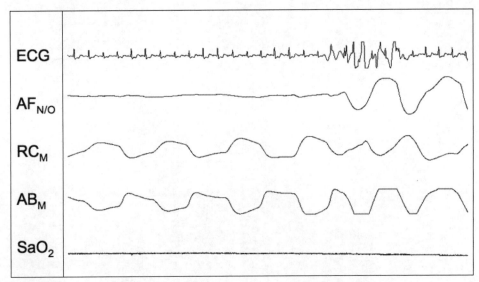

Figure 28.

SECTION 2

Answers

1. Answer: B

EDUCATIONAL OBJECTIVE: Compare the sleep architecture among the elderly with that among young adults.

EXPLANATION: Compared to younger adults, sleep in older adults is characterized by longer latencies to sleep onset and increased wake time after sleep onset (WASO). The duration of nighttime awakenings is also increased. Older adults have more sleep stage shifts and reduced total sleep time, sleep efficiency, and N3 or slow-wave sleep (SWS). The percentage of stage REM sleep is also decreased in persons over 50 years of age. Normal aging is associated with decreased homeostatic sleep drive, decreased arousal threshold, and increased frequency of daytime napping. In addition, older adults have increased prevalence of sleep disorders, such as insomnia, obstructive sleep apnea, and periodic limb movement disorder.

Reference:

Harrington JJ, Lee-Chiong T. Sleep and older patients. *Clin Chest Med.* 2007; 28:673–684.

2. Answer: D

EDUCATIONAL OBJECTIVE: Identify the characteristic features of sleep paralysis.

EXPLANATION: Sleep paralysis is a temporary inability to move that occurs at sleep onset or upon awakening from sleep. It is experienced by approximately 40% to 80% of persons with narcolepsy but can occasionally occur in otherwise healthy persons after sleep deprivation, irregular sleep patterns, or alcohol ingestion.

These episodes can be very frightening. Patients often describe feelings of impending doom or suffocation, and auditory or tactile hallucinations can occur. During an episode, patients are unable to speak or move their limbs but they may report full or partial awareness. Events usually last a few minutes and either end spontaneously or after external stimulation, such as a touch or noise. Recovery is immediate and full. Because of the often disturbing nature of these episodes, upsetting memories can be long lasting.

References:

1. American Academy of Sleep Medicine. *International Classification of Sleep Disorders: Diagnostic and Coding Manual.* 2nd ed. Westchester, Ill: American Academy of Sleep Medicine; 2005:81–86
2. Nielsen TA, Zadra A. Nightmares and other common dream disturbances. In: Kryger MH, Roth T, Dement WC, eds. *Principles and Practice of Sleep Medicine.* 4th ed. Philadelphia, Pa: Elsevier Saunders; 2005:926–930

3. Answer: C

EDUCATIONAL OBJECTIVE: Describe the mechanism of action of caffeine.

EXPLANATION: Caffeine is classified as a methylxanthine. It is the most widely consumed stimulant and is found in a variety of products, such as coffee, tea, soda, and chocolate. Adenosine is a central nervous system (CNS) neurotransmitter that promotes slow-wave sleep. Levels of adenosine rise throughout continuous wakefulness and decrease during recovery sleep. Caffeine exerts its alerting effects primarily via antagonism of A1 adenosine receptors on neurons located in the basal forebrain. Caffeine ingestion is associated with objective findings of increased sleep latency and decreased total sleep time, as well as increased stage N1 sleep, and decreases in N3 and REM sleep.

Caffeine can improve alertness and cognitive performance and decrease both subjective and objective sleepiness during sleep deprivation. Usual dosages of caffeine range from 50 to 200 mg. Ingestion of higher dosages (up to 600 mg) in sustained-release forms may give rise to levels of alertness approaching that of lower-dose stimulants. The development of tolerance, however, limits the effectiveness of caffeine as therapy for disorders of chronic hypersomnolence. Caffeine's half-life is usually 3 to 5 hours. Common side effects include nausea, diarrhea, muscle twitching, cramps, and insomnia. Headaches, excessive sleepiness, and irritability may develop after abrupt withdrawal.

Reference:

Nishino S, Mignot E. Wake-promoting medications: basic mechanisms and pharmacology. In: Kryger MH, Roth T, Dement WC, eds. *Principles and Practice of Sleep Medicine.* 4th ed. Philadelphia, Pa: Elsevier Saunders; 2005:468–483.

4. Answer: D

EDUCATIONAL OBJECTIVE: Identify polysomnographic features associated with the intake of selective serotonin reuptake inhibitors (SSRIs).

EXPLANATION: SSRIs include sertraline, citalopram, fluvoxamine, fluoxetine, citalopram, and paroxetine. Insomnia and daytime sedation are reported side effects of specific SSRIs. Paroxetine and fluvoxamine are among the most sedating of the SSRIs. SSRIs may worsen periodic limb movements of sleep and symptoms of restless legs syndrome. Common polysomnographic features associated with these medications include increases in sleep latency, nighttime awakenings and wake time after sleep onset (WASO), and decreases in sleep efficiency and total sleep time. These medications tend to suppress REM sleep and may disrupt motor inhibition during this stage of sleep. The epoch in this question demonstrates a commonly observed artifact associated with fluoxetine use, namely increased eye movements during NREM sleep, or "Prozac eyes."

5. Answer: B

EDUCATIONAL OBJECTIVE: Describe the characteristic findings associated with sleep-related groaning.

EXPLANATION: Sleep-related groaning or catathrenia is characterized by repetitive expiratory moaning or groaning during sleep. These episodes typically occur in clusters during the second half of the night and are noted principally during stage REM sleep. Polysomnography generally demonstrates normal sleep architecture. An electroencephalographic (EEG) arousal frequently denotes the end of an episode. Epileptiform discharges are not associated with this condition. Prevalence is unknown but it appears to be very rare with a male predominance. There is no reported association with pulmonary or psychiatric conditions. Bed partners or roommates often initiate clinical evaluation since affected patients are often asymptomatic or report nonspecific complaints, such as restless sleep or daytime fatigue. Physical examination is usually unremarkable. Course tends to chronic.

Reference:

American Academy of Sleep Medicine. *International Classification of Sleep Disorders: Diagnostic and Coding Manual.* 2nd ed. Westchester, Ill: American Academy of Sleep Medicine; 2005:165–167.

6. Answer: B

EDUCATIONAL OBJECTIVE: Describe the anatomic and functional differences between Frédérick Bremer's different cat preparations (i.e., encéphale isolé and cerveau isolé).

EXPLANATION: Frédérick Bremer was a neurophysiologist who in the mid-1930s reported the findings of his innovative cat transection experiments. In the cerveau isolé preparation, a mesencephalic transection was performed just behind the origin of the third nerve nuclei. This resulted in features of persistent electroencephalographic (EEG) sleep characteristics as well as progressive miosis. Bremer's encéphale isolé preparation, on the other hand, involved transection at the level of the lower medulla and resulted in EEG features of alternating sleep and wake phases. As these investigations were conducted prior to the groundbreaking discovery by Moruzzi and Magoun of the brainstem reticular activating system, Bremer initially concluded that these findings supported a passive theory of sleep or cortical "deafferentation."

References:

1. Kerkhofs M, Lavie P. Frédérick Bremer 1892–1982: a pioneer in sleep research. *Sleep Med Rev.* 2000; 4(5):505–514.
2. Dement WC. History of sleep physiology and medicine. In: Kryger MH, Roth T, Dement WC, eds. *Principles and Practice of Sleep Medicine.* 4th ed. Philadelphia, Pa: Elsevier Saunders; 2005:1–12.

7. Answer: B

EDUCATIONAL OBJECTIVE: Describe reported findings of cerebral positron emission tomography (PET) imaging studies in patients with insomnia.

EXPLANATION: Nofzinger et al. have utilized [^{18}F]-fluorodeoxyglucose (FDG) PET imaging to assess cerebral metabolism in subjects with insomnia. In a comparison study of regional metabolic differences between a small sample of insomniacs and healthy controls, those with insomnia demonstrated relative hypometabolism in the prefrontal cortex during wakefulness. This study also suggested increased whole brain metabolism across waking and sleep states. In a more recent study, relative hypermetabolism was noted in certain brain regions during NREM sleep that was associated with increased subjective and objective wake time after sleep onset (WASO).

References:

1. Nofzinger EA, Buysse DJ. Functional neuroimaging evidence for hyperarousal in insomnia. *Am J Psychiatry.* 2004; 161:2126–2129.
2. Nofzinger EA, Nissen C, Germain A, et al. Regional cerebral metabolic correlates of WASO during NREM sleep in insomnia. *J Clin Sleep Med.* 2006; 2(3):316–322.

8. Answer: D

EDUCATIONAL OBJECTIVE: Understand the clinical features associated with the development of restless legs syndrome (RLS) augmentation related to dopaminergic therapy.

EXPLANATION: RLS is a disorder characterized by an urge to move the limbs and is accompanied by unpleasant or uncomfortable sensations. These sensations are worse during periods of rest or inactivity and are, at least partially, lessened with movement. Symptoms are worse, or occur only, during the evening or night. Augmentation is a complication associated with dopaminergic therapy for RLS. Clinical features of augmentation include symptoms that 1) occur earlier in the evening or day (at least 2 hours before what was experienced prior to dopaminergic initiation), 2) are increased in severity, 3) display a shorter latency to onset during restful periods, 4) extend to previously unaffected body parts, and 5) require dosage escalation or change in therapy. Augmentation is more commonly associated with levodopa therapy but may be seen, although less frequently, in patients taking dopamine agonists. Rebound is related to withdrawal symptoms that typically occur later in the nocturnal sleep period when L-dopa is administered at bedtime.

References:

1. Paulus W, Trenkwalder C. Less is more: pathophysiology of dopaminergic-therapy-related augmentation in restless legs syndrome. *Lancet Neurol.* 2006; 5:878–886.
2. Montplaisir J, Allen RP, Walters AS, et al. Restless legs syndrome and periodic limb movements during sleep. In: Kryger MH, Roth T, Dement WC, eds. *Principles and Practice of Sleep Medicine.* 4th ed. Philadelphia, Pa: Elsevier Saunders; 2005:839–852.

9. Answer: D

EDUCATIONAL OBJECTIVE: Describe the characteristic features of monoamine oxidase inhibitors (MAOIs) on sleep and sleep architecture.

EXPLANATION: MAOIs inhibit enzymes that metabolize dopamine, serotonin, and norepinephrine. The classic MAOIs, which include isocarboxazid, tranylcypromine, and phenelzine, irreversibly inhibit MAO-A and MAO-B enzymes. Reported side effects include either daytime sedation or insomnia. Polysomnographic features consist of decreased total sleep time and marked reduction in stage REM sleep. These older MAOIs are regarded as the most potent REM sleep suppressants. Rebound REM sleep can occur upon drug withdrawal. Newer MAOIs, such as moclobemide and brofaromine, reversibly and selectively inhibit the MAO-A enzyme. Although sleep disturbance and insomnia have been reported with these newer agents, no significant alteration in REM sleep has been noted.

Reference:

Schweitzer PK. Drugs that disturb sleep and wakefulness. In: Kryger MH, Roth T, Dement WC, eds. *Principles and Practice of Sleep Medicine.* 4th ed. Philadelphia, Pa: Elsevier Saunders; 2005:499–518.

10. Answer: B

EDUCATIONAL OBJECTIVE: Describe sleep-related features that are associated with lithium carbonate use.

EXPLANATION: Lithium carbonate is primarily prescribed for the treatment of bipolar disorder (i.e., manic depression). Lithium can produce hypersomnolence despite improved subjective nocturnal sleep, as well as deficits in cognitive and psychomotor performance. Polysomnographic findings may include decreased stage N1 sleep and increased stages N2 and N3 sleep. REM sleep disturbance is not uniform but typically includes prolonged REM sleep latency and decreased REM sleep. REM sleep rebound may be associated with abrupt lithium withdrawal.

Reference:

Schweitzer PK. Drugs that disturb sleep and wakefulness. In: Kryger MH, Roth T, Dement WC, eds. *Principles and Practice of Sleep Medicine.* 4th ed. Philadelphia, Pa: Elsevier Saunders; 2005:499–518.

11. Answer: B

EDUCATIONAL OBJECTIVE: Understand the adjunctive use of modafinil therapy for symptoms of residual excessive daytime sleepiness in obstructive sleep apnea (OSA).

EXPLANATION: Modafinil is a novel wake-promoting agent that differs chemically and pharmacologically from other stimulant medications. The American Academy of Sleep Medicine (AASM) lists adjunctive modafinil treatment as a standard recommendation for patients with OSA who report symptoms of residual daytime sleepiness despite effective positive airway pressure (PAP) therapy, provided there are no other known causes (e.g., another sleep disorder, poor sleep hygiene, insufficient sleep) of hypersomnia. Partial attenuation of residual daytime sleepiness after modafinil administration was noted in studies included in the AASM review. Nightly nasal continuous positive airway pressure (CPAP) usage with adjuvant modafinil treatment varied across studies and remained either unchanged or mildly, although significantly, decreased. Nocturnal sleep parameters did not differ significantly between modafinil-treated subjects and controls.

References:

1. Morgenthaler TI, Kapen S, Lee-Chiong T, et al. Obstructive sleep apnea. Practice parameters for the medical therapy of obstructive sleep apnea. *SLEEP* 2006; 29(8):1031–1035.
2. Roth T, Schwartz J, Hirshkowitz M, et al. Evaluation of the safety of modafinil for treatment of excessive sleepiness. *J Clin Sleep Med.* 2007; 3(6):595–602.

12. Answer: A

EDUCATIONAL OBJECTIVE: Identify the common diagnostic features of Kleine–Levin syndrome.

EXPLANATION: Kleine–Levin syndrome is one form of recurrent hypersomnia. Affected individuals have recurrent episodes of excessive sleepiness that lasts from a few days to several weeks in duration. Patients may sleep for prolonged periods, 16 or more hours per day, and may also demonstrate cognitive and behavioral abnormalities. Binge eating, hypersexuality, disinhibition, and weight gain have been reported. Between hypersomnia occurrences, patients exhibit normal sleep, behavior, and cognitive functioning. The typical age of onset is during early adolescence and the condition is more prevalent in males. The course is generally benign and episodes tend to diminish in frequency, severity, and duration with time.

Reference:

American Academy of Sleep Medicine. *International Classification of Sleep Disorders: Diagnostic and Coding Manual.* 2nd ed. Westchester, Ill: American Academy of Sleep Medicine; 2005:95–97.

13. Answer: C

EDUCATIONAL OBJECTIVE: Describe the characteristic features of sleep-related eating disorder (SRED).

EXPLANATION: SRED is characterized by recurrent arousals from the main sleep period associated with involuntary eating and drinking. This condition is often associated with a prior history of sleepwalking but other sleep disorders are not uncommon. Although individuals typically have only partial recall of these nocturnal events, others may report substantial alertness or complete unawareness. Patients may describe the consumption of high-caloric and peculiar food. Inappropriate (e.g., raw or frozen) foods or toxic substances may also be ingested. Alcoholic intake during these episodes is rare. Other consequences associated with this condition include sleep-related injury associated with hazardous behaviors or activities conducted during episodes, sleep disturbance, and morning anorexia. Females are more commonly affected. This disorder should be distinguished from nocturnal eating syndrome (NES). Symptoms of NES include overeating that occurs after the regular evening meal and prior to sleep onset. In contrast to SRED, persons with NES are fully awake during overeating episodes, foods consumed are typical, and abnormal or strange behaviors are absent.

References:

1. American Academy of Sleep Medicine. *International Classification of Sleep Disorders: Diagnostic and Coding Manual.* 2nd ed. Westchester, Ill: American Academy of Sleep Medicine; 2005:173–175.
2. Benca RM, Schenck CH. Sleep and eating disorders. In: Kryger MH, Roth T, Dement WC, eds. *Principles and Practice of Sleep Medicine.* 4th ed. Philadelphia, Pa: Elsevier Saunders; 2005:1341–1344.

14. Answer: A

EDUCATIONAL OBJECTIVE: Understand basic techniques of chronotherapy for circadian rhythm sleep disorders.

EXPLANATION: Traditional chronotherapy for delayed sleep phase syndrome (DSPS) involves successively delaying bedtimes by 3 hours per day until the bedtime approximates an appropriate, or socially acceptable time for the patient. Alternatively, modified chronotherapy requires one night of total sleep deprivation followed by an advanced sleep time, usually in increments of 90 minutes. This schedule is repeated until an appropriate bedtime is achieved. Strict adherence to the resultant sleep–wake schedule is necessary since patients may revert quickly back to their prior delayed sleep–wake rhythm. Chronotherapy aimed at treating persons with advanced sleep phase syndrome progressively advances bedtimes but reversions occur quickly.

Reference:

Lee-Chiong T, Harrington J. Circadian rhythm sleep disorders, delayed sleep phase type (delayed sleep phase disorder): treatment using chronotherapy. In: *Case Book of Sleep Medicine: A Learning Companion to the International Classification of Sleep Disorders.* 2nd ed. (ICSD-2). Westchester, Ill: American Academy of Sleep Medicine; 2008:204–206.

15. Answer: A

EDUCATIONAL OBJECTIVE: Identify clinical and polysomnographic features of alcohol abstinence.

EXPLANATION: Sleep disturbances are commonly reported with alcohol use, withdrawal, and abstinence. During the first few weeks of abstinence, various sleep measures are typically disturbed and include increased stage REM sleep, sleep latency, and wake time after sleep onset (WASO). Total sleep time tends to gradually improve over time. However, increase in stage REM sleep percentage may persist for up to 1 or more years after cessation of alcohol use. Although not consistent across all studies, there is some evidence to suggest that one or more REM sleep measures, including shortened REM sleep latency as well as increased REM sleep percentage and REM density, may be predictive of short-term relapse. In terms of long-term relapse, however, prolonged baseline sleep latency (both objective and subjective) is a better predictor than other sleep measures.

References:

1. Drummond S, Gillin J, Smith T, et al. The sleep of abstinent pure primary alcoholic patients: natural course and relationship to relapse. *Alcohol Clin Exp Res.* 1998; 22(8):1796–1802.
2. Kirk J, Brower MD, Michael S, et al. Insomnia, self-medication, and relapse to alcoholism. *Am J Psychiatry.* 2001; 158:399–404.
3. Brower KJ, Aldrich MS, Hall JM. Polysomnographic and subjective sleep predictors of alcoholic relapse. *Alcohol Clin Exp Res.* 1998; 22(8):1864–1871.

16. Answer: D

EDUCATIONAL OBJECTIVE: Describe the clinical features associated with inadequate sleep hygiene.

EXPLANATION: Inadequate sleep hygiene is a disorder characterized by insomnia that lasts for at least 1 month. In addition, individuals with this condition must also describe one or more practices or behaviors that are nonconducive to the maintenance of a regular sleep–wake schedule. Examples of sleep-disturbing practices include 1) improper or varying sleep schedules, excessive napping, or spending prolonged time in bed; 2) ingestion of substances that may interfere with sleep onset or maintenance, such as caffeine or nicotine, close to bedtime; 3) engaging in activities that are too alerting or stimulating close to bedtime; 4) engaging in activities in bed that are not related to sleep or intimacy, such as watching television or studying; or 5) sleeping in an uncomfortable environment.

This patient's symptoms are not consistent with a diagnosis of delayed sleep phase syndrome because his sleep normalizes when he refrains from using electronic devices. Psychophysiologic insomnia is not likely since he typically falls asleep quickly at home when not engaging in other activities. He also does not report symptoms suggestive of conditioned arousal. Environmental sleep disorder is a condition marked by one or more factors that disturb sleep onset or maintenance; removal of the responsible irritant usually results in resolution of the sleep complaint.

17. Answer: A

EDUCATIONAL OBJECTIVE: Describe clinical features of the circadian rhythm sleep disorder, free-running type.

EXPLANATION: Circadian rhythm sleep disorder, free-running (nonentrained) type, is a condition marked by circadian pacemaker oscillations that are slightly longer than 24 hours and that are not entrained by environmental time cues. This results in a characteristic sleep–wake period that progressively delays over time. Individuals report symptoms of insomnia or daytime sleepiness and impaired daytime functioning, along with a progressive delay in sleep times. The vast majority of persons affected are totally blind; however, cases in sighted individuals do occur but are rare. The pathogenesis among blind persons is thought to be related to a marked reduction or absence of photic stimulation to the circadian pacemaker. In sighted persons, psychiatric and neurologic disorders are often associated. Sleep logs, with or without actigraphy, preferably conducted for 7 or more days, typically depict sleep–wake times that are progressively delayed. Low-dose melatonin is frequently prescribed for all patients and is taken near the estimated dim-light melatonin onset (DLMO) only after sleep–wake times have drifted to a more socially appropriate schedule. Bright light therapy may be considered in patients with light responsiveness.

References:

1. American Academy of Sleep Medicine. *International Classification of Sleep Disorders: Diagnostic and Coding Manual.* 2nd ed. Westchester, Ill: American Academy of Sleep Medicine; 2005:126–128.
2. Sack R, Auckley D, Auger RR, et al. Circadian rhythm sleep disorders: Part II, Advanced sleep phase disorder, delayed sleep phase disorder, free-running disorder, and irregular sleep–wake rhythm. An American Academy of Sleep Medicine Review. *Sleep.* 2007; 30(11):1484–1501.

18. Answer: A

EDUCATIONAL OBJECTIVE: Describe the distinguishing clinical features of irregular sleep–wake rhythm (ISWR).

EXPLANATION: The prominent features of the circadian rhythm sleep disorder ISWR, collected from sleep log or actigraphy data, include sleep–wake cycles that do not have an apparent circadian pattern, absence of a prominent sleep period, and multiple (i.e., three or more) sleep bouts of differing duration. However, in spite of these derangements, total 24-hour sleep duration commonly remains age appropriate. Patients often describe chronic symptoms of insomnia and/or daytime sleepiness. The etiology of this circadian dysrhythmia is unclear but its association with central nervous system (CNS) injury and neurodegenerative disorders, such as dementia, is commonly noted. Institutionalized patients and other individuals who may have decreased exposure to zeitgebers (e.g., sunlight, physical activity, or social interaction) may be more susceptible. Studies utilizing a variety of interventions such as bright light therapy and environmental changes, have reported modest, but inconsistent results. Melatonin may be considered in children with severe neurologic deficits.

References:

1. Sack R, Auckley D, Auger RR, et al. Circadian rhythm sleep disorders: Part II, Advanced sleep phase disorder, delayed sleep phase disorder, free-running disorder, and irregular sleep–wake rhythm. An American Academy of Sleep Medicine Review. *Sleep.* 2007; 30(11):1484–1501.
2. American Academy of Sleep Medicine. *International Classification of Sleep Disorders: Diagnostic and Coding Manual.* 2nd ed. Westchester, Ill: American Academy of Sleep Medicine; 2005:124–125.

19. Answer: A

EDUCATIONAL OBJECTIVE: Identify genetic syndromes that may predispose to the development of obstructive sleep apnea (OSA) in children.

EXPLANATION: Down syndrome (trisomy 21) is a disorder that is characterized by several craniofacial features that may predispose to OSA. These include mid-facial and mandibular hypoplasia, macroglossia, micrognathia, highly arched and narrow palates, and relative adenotonsillar enlargement. Muscular hypotonia and obesity may also result in increased upper airway collapsibility in these patients. Other genetic syndromes, such as Treacher Collins and Pierre Robin sequence, are associated with mandibular hypoplasia that leads to tongue base encroachment into the upper airway. Maxillary hypoplasia, noted in craniosynostoses (e.g., Apert and Crouzon syndromes), may lead to upper airway obstruction due to a posterior repositioning of the palate into the nasopharynx. Prader–Willi syndrome is marked by obesity, minor upper airway narrowing, hyperphagia, hypotonia, short stature, hypogonadism, as well as behavioral abnormalities and developmental delay. OSA is commonly noted in these children as well.

References:

1. Wills LM, Swift JQ, Moller KT. Craniofacial syndromes in sleep disorders. In: Lee-Chiong TL, ed. *Sleep: A Comprehensive Handbook.* Hoboken, NJ: Wiley; 2006.
2. Lee-Chiong T. *Sleep Medicine: Essentials and Review.* USA: Oxford University Press; 2008.

20. Answer: A

EDUCATIONAL OBJECTIVE: Understand common sleep-related abnormalities in blind persons.

EXPLANATION: Blind persons tend to report more sleep complaints than sighted individuals. Leger et al. found a higher prevalence and severity of insomnia as well as free-running circadian rhythms among blind subjects. Although a free-running circadian disorder is common in totally blind persons with an estimated prevalence of 18% to 50%, insomnia remains more prevalent. Blind persons, even without conscious or unconscious light perception, do not always demonstrate an unsynchronized circadian rhythm, suggesting that other factors, such as an endogenous circadian pacemaker oscillation very near to a 24-hour cycle or other nonphotic time cues, may be present in these individuals. Melatonin has been evaluated as an entrainment therapy for circadian rhythm abnormalities in blind patients. Several studies have demonstrated its effectiveness but the time of administration is important to avoid continued free-running.

References:

1. Sack RL, Lewy AJ, Blood ML, et al. Circadian rhythm abnormalities in totally blind people: incidence and clinical significance. *J Clin Endocrinol Metab.* 1992; 75:127–133.
2. Leger D, Guilleminault C, Santos C, et al. Prevalence of sleep/wake disorders in persons with blindness. *Clin Sci.* 1999; 97:193–199.
3. American Academy of Sleep Medicine. *International Classification of Sleep Disorders: Diagnostic and Coding Manual.* 2nd ed. Westchester, Ill: American Academy of Sleep Medicine; 2005:126–128.

21. Answer: D

EDUCATIONAL OBJECTIVE: Identify the features of a paced cardiac rhythm.

EXPLANATION: These electroencephalographic (EGG) samples (A: 15-second epoch; B: 5-second epoch) exhibit a paced cardiac rhythm. Note the pace spike preceding each QRS complex. Part A (Fig. 2) also demonstrates a premature ventricular contraction.

22. Answer: D

EDUCATIONAL OBJECTIVE: Identify the central nervous system structure that releases the neurotransmitter histamine.

EXPLANATION: The tuberomammillary nucleus of the posterior hypothalamus, which projects to the forebrain, releases the neurotransmitter histamine. During wakefulness, the discharge rates of the neurons located in the tuberomammillary nucleus increase. First-generation histamine-1 antagonists, such as chlorpheniramine and diphenhydramine, are lipophilic compounds that readily cross the blood–brain barrier and can cause sedation and daytime sleepiness. For this reason, they are commonly used as over-the-counter sleep aids. Newer, or second-generation, hydrophilic histamine-1 antagonists, such as certirizine, fexofenadine, and loratadine, do not easily cross the blood–brain barrier and are, therefore, less likely to cause sedation at their usual prescribed dosages.

Reference:

Lee-Chiong T. *Sleep Medicine: Essentials and Review.* USA: Oxford University Press; 2008.

23. Answer: A

EDUCATIONAL OBJECTIVE: Understand what constitutes REM sleep latency on multiple sleep latency tests (MSLTs).

EXPLANATION: Stage REM sleep is characterized by electroencephalographic (EEG) "desynchronization" (i.e., low-voltage theta and beta waves), muscle atonia (dampened chin and limb electromyography [EMG]), and rapid eye movements (bursts of saccadic ocular movements recorded on electrooculography [EOG]). EEG activity resembling "saw tooth" waves may be present (see Fig. 3). Sleep-onset REM periods (SOREMPs) are scored during an MSLT nap period when polysomnography (PSG) meets criteria for stage REM sleep occupying greater than 50% of any 30-second epoch of sleep. Sleep latency for a clinical MSLT is determined by the first epoch of sleep (any stage) from "lights out." REM sleep latency is the time between sleep onset and the first REM sleep epoch (regardless of intervening wakefulness).

In the above scenario, REM sleep latency would correspond to the duration from sleep onset (10:15 a.m.) to the first epoch of REM sleep (10:18 a.m.), or 3 minutes (assuming, of course, that no other epochs of stage REM sleep occurred between these two time points). Naps are terminated when one of the following occurs: 1) no sleep is recorded after 20 minutes; 2) 15 minutes after sleep onset; 3) or unequivocal stage REM sleep is noted.

24. Answer: A

EDUCATIONAL OBJECTIVE: Understand the genetic, pathologic, and clinical features of fatal familial insomnia (FFI).

EXPLANATION: FFI is a rare autosomonal dominant disorder. This disease is characterized by progressive sleep loss, autonomic hyperactivity, and neurologic and motor disturbances. The typical age of onset is between 36 and 62 years. There is no gender predilection. Most patients present with symptoms of cognitive disturbances in vigilance and memory, as well as sleep loss. Autonomic dysregulatory symptoms (e.g., pyrexia, tachycardia, tachypnea, and hypertension) are also reported. Motor and neurologic abnormalities often include myoclonus, dysarthria, pyramidal signs, tremors, diplopia, dysphagia, and sphincter incontinence. Death, often a result of complications of infection, occurs within 8 to 72 months of diagnosis. The hereditary form of this disease is secondary to GAC to AAC point mutation at the 178 codon of the *PRNP* gene located on chromosome 20. This mutation cosegregates with a methionine (Met) polymorphism at codon 129. Methionine–methionine homozygosity at codon 129 is associated with a more rapid disease progression (mean survival of 9 months), while a methionine–valine heterozygosity is generally related to a longer disease duration (mean survival of 31 months). A sporadic form, which lacks the above-noted PRNP mutations, has been reported. Neuropathologic investigations have demonstrated severe neuronal atrophy and astrogliosis in the anterior ventral and dorsomedial thalamic nuclei. The inferior olivary nuclei are also similarly affected.

References:

1. Montagna P. Fatal familial insomnia: a model disease in sleep physiopathology. *Sleep Med Rev.* 2005; 9:339–353.
2. American Academy of Sleep Medicine. *International Classification of Sleep Disorders: Diagnostic and Coding Manual.* 2nd ed. Westchester, Ill: American Academy of Sleep Medicine; 2005:226–228.

25. Answer: C

EDUCATIONAL OBJECTIVE: Describe the electroencephalographic features and primary neuroanatomic generator of sleep spindles.

EXPLANATION: Sleep spindles are short trains of oscillating fusiform activity with a frequency of 12 to 14 Hz and an amplitude typically less than 50 μV (20 to 100 μV). They are most prominent in the central derivations. Although maximal during stage N2 sleep, these waveforms can be identified in stage N3 sleep but are not, by definition, seen in stage N1 sleep. The presence of sleep spindles and K-complexes, in part, distinguishes stage N1 from stage N2 sleep.

Sleep spindles are generated in the thalamic reticular (RE) nucleus. The exact mechanism of spindle generation has not been completely elucidated, but discharges from RE nuclei during prolonged hyperpolarization are postulated to be involved in the initiation of sleep spindles. Spindles are transferred, via thalamocortical neurons, to the cerebral cortex, where synchronization and propagation occur.

26. Answer: D

EDUCATIONAL OBJECTIVE: Describe circadian patterns of gastric acid secretion.

EXPLANATION: Basal gastric acid secretion demonstrates a noticeable circadian rhythmicity. Acid secretion is maximal between 10 p.m. and 2 a.m. and is minimal in the morning hours between 5 a.m. and 11 a.m. Whether basal gastric acid secretion is altered because of sleep per se is not clear. Other upper gastroesophageal physiologic changes related to sleep include diminished swallowing, salivation, and esophageal motility. These features may predispose to nocturnal gastroesophageal reflux and prolonged mucosal acid contact.

27. Answer: C

EDUCATIONAL OBJECTIVE: Recognize the clinical features of congenital central alveolar hypoventilation syndrome (CCHS).

EXPLANATION: CCHS is a rare disorder usually affecting newborns and infants, which is characterized by hypoventilation due to a failure of autonomic central breathing control mechanisms. Hypoventilation is most pronounced during sleep (particularly NREM sleep) and is related to impaired central chemoreceptor responsiveness to hypercapnia and hypoxia. Hypoventilation is not the result of another cardiopulmonary, neuromuscular, or metabolic disorder. The pathophysiology of this condition is unknown but recent evidence supports the association of a de novo mutation in the *PHOX2B* gene in the vast majority of cases. Although most patients with severe disease require mechanically assisted ventilation during sleep (when hypoventilation is worse), most do not need ventilatory support during wakefulness. Syndrome presentation is variable but patients typically have observed shallow, irregular breathing and periods of apneas. Other associated disturbances may include neural crest tumors, swallowing and feeding difficulties, autonomic dysfunction, and aganglionic megacolon (Hirschsprung disease). If adequate ventilatory assistance is provided, long-term consequences of severe hypoventilation, such as cor pulmonale, mental retardation, and seizures, may be ameliorated.

References:

1. American Academy of Sleep Medicine. *International Classification of Sleep Disorders: Diagnostic and Coding Manual.* 2nd ed. Westchester, Ill: American Academy of Sleep Medicine; 2005:63–65.
2. Amiel J, Laudier B, Attié-Bitach T, et al. Polyalanine expansion and frameshift mutations of the paired-like homeobox gene PHOX2B in congenital central hypoventilation syndrome. *Nat Genet.* 2003; 33(4):459–461.
3. Casey KR, Cantillo KO, Brown LK, et al. Sleep-related hypoventilation/hypoxemic syndromes. *Chest.* 2007; 131(6):1936–1948 (Review).

28. Answer: A

EDUCATIONAL OBJECTIVE: Describe the effects of sleep deprivation on antibody response to vaccination.

EXPLANATION: Antibody response to immunization after a period of sleep restriction or deprivation has been evaluated in only a few small clinical trials. In one study, antibody response to hepatitis A (HAV) vaccination was evaluated after one night of total sleep deprivation that occurred immediately following immunization. This study found significantly lower HAV antibody levels at 4 weeks. In another study, the effect of chronic partial sleep restriction on antibody production after influenza vaccination was investigated. Titers of IgG antibody were assessed at baseline, 10 days, and 21 to 30 days post vaccination. Although mean antibody titers were significantly decreased at 10 days after vaccination compared to normal controls, they did not differ significantly between groups during the plateau phase. Further, passively immunized mice did not demonstrate increased IgG anti-influenza catabolism after sleep deprivation. In a more recent trial, persons with untreated moderate to severe obstructive sleep apnea and healthy controls received influenza vaccination. Immune responsiveness was not different between groups and did not correlate with apnea severity, sleepiness, or sleep disruption.

References:

1. Lange T, Perras B, Fehm HL, et al. Sleep enhances the human antibody response to hepatitis A vaccination. *Psychosom Med.* 2003; 65:831–835.
2. Spiegel K, Sheridan JF, Van Cauter E. Effect of sleep deprivation on response to immunization. *JAMA.* 2002; 288(12):1471–1472.

3. Renegar KB, Floyd R, Krueger JM. Effect of sleep deprivation on serum influenza-specific IgG. *Sleep.* 1998; 21(1):19–24.

4. Dopp JM, Wiegert NA, Moran JJ, et al. Humoral immune responses to influenza vaccination in patients with obstructive sleep apnea. *Pharmacotherapy.* 2007; 27(11):1483–1489.

29. Answer: B

EDUCATIONAL OBJECTIVE: Identify characteristic features of the cardioballistic artifact.

EXPLANATION: This 30-second epoch demonstrates an aberration in the airflow channel consistent with cardiogenic oscillations (sometimes referred to as "cardioballistic artifact"). These oscillations are thought to represent a "pulse" wave, as they correspond temporally to cardiac contractions and electrocardiographic (ECG) tracings. These pulsations may lead to similar waveforms in the electroencephalographic (EEG) channels due to body and head movements. These oscillations are often recorded during both exhalation and central apneic events and can occur in both airway and effort channels. Whether these oscillations are indicative of upper airway patency has not been clearly established. Some investigators have suggested that these findings may be useful in distinguishing central from obstructive apneas.

References:

1. Ayappa I, Norman RG, Rapoport DM, et al. Cardiogenic oscillations on the airflow signal during continuous positive airway pressure as a marker of central apnea. *Chest.* 1999; 116:660–666.

2. Morrell MJ, Badr MS, Harms CA, et al. The assessment of upper airway patency during apnea using cardiogenic oscillations in the airflow signal. *Sleep.* 1995; 18(8):651–658.

30. Answer: D

EDUCATIONAL OBJECTIVE: Recognize the clinical features of restless legs syndrome (RLS).

EXPLANATION: RLS is a common disorder, affecting about 10% of the population. It is a clinical diagnosis made by patient history and physical examination. Four criteria are necessary to make the diagnosis of RLS, namely, uncomfortable sensation giving rise to a desire to move the legs; motor restlessness; symptoms having a circadian rhythmicity that are worse in the evening or at night as well as at rest; and relief by activity. Periodic leg movements in sleep are not necessary to make a diagnosis of RLS. Differential diagnoses include hypnic jerks or sleep starts, fragmentary myoclonus, painful leg and moving toes, paresthesia due to neuropathy, nocturnal leg cramps, and neuroleptic-induced akathisia that is characterized by total body restlessness. Akathisia is not worse at rest and has no circadian rhythmicity.

Reference:

Kushida CA. Clinical presentation, diagnosis, and quality of life issues in restless legs syndrome. *Am J Med.* 2007; 120(1A):S4–S12.

31. Answer: B

EDUCATIONAL OBJECTIVE: Identify the various conditions associated with restless legs syndrome (RLS).

EXPLANATION: RLS can be either primary or associated with secondary causes. Primary RLS is hereditary. An autosomal dominant mode of inheritance has been described in some families. It is characterized by an earlier age of onset (<45 years) and slowly progressive symptoms. In contrast, secondary RLS is characterized by more rapid progression of symptoms and later age of onset. Secondary causes of RLS include iron deficiency anemia, renal failure, and pregnancy. These conditions share in common a defect in iron metabolism. Serum ferritin <50µg/L warrants iron supplementation even in absence of significant anemia since ferritin serves as an iron storage protein as well as an iron transporter. Low cerebrospinal fluid (CSF) ferritin levels and decreased brain iron levels have also been found in patients with RLS. Severity of RLS is worsened by low levels of serum ferritin, and iron supplementation decreases RLS symptoms.

32. Answer: C

EDUCATIONAL OBJECTIVE: Recognize the medications that can exacerbate restless legs syndrome (RLS).

EXPLANATION: RLS symptoms can be exacerbated by dopamine-blocking agents, antidepressants, including selective serotonin reuptake inhibitors (SSRIs) and tricyclic antidepressants (TCAs), antihistamines, and lithium. Pharmacologic and clinical studies suggest a close relationship between iron, dopamine, and RLS. Iron is a cofactor for tyrosine hydroxylase, a critical enzyme for dopamine synthesis. Decreased quantity of iron has been demonstrated in the brain of subjects with RLS and could alter dopaminergic function. Dopamine and iron levels fall at night, indicating a circadian pattern. RLS improves with the use of dopamine agonists and is worsened by dopamine blockers, further supporting a role for dopamine in the physiopathology of RLS.

SSRIs increase serotonin transmission, which leads to inhibition of the function of dopaminergic neurons. Neuroleptics are dopamine-blocking agents. Lithium has been shown to decrease dopamine release.

References:

1. Ryan M, Slevin JT. Restless legs syndrome. *Am J Health Syst Pharm.* 2006; 63:1599–1612.
2. Allen RP. Controversies and challenges in defining the etiology and pathophysiology of restless legs syndrome. *Am J Med.* 2007; 120(1A):S13–S21.

33. Answer: B

EDUCATIONAL OBJECTIVE: Identify the effects of alcohol on sleep.

EXPLANATION: Acute alcohol intoxication has been associated with decreased sleep latency, reduced total REM sleep, prolonged REM sleep latency, increased NREM sleep, reduced sleep efficiency, and sleep disruption. Even a low dose of alcohol has been shown to reduce REM sleep in healthy subjects. Alcohol can also worsen sleep-disordered breathing.

Reference:

Miyata S, Noda A, Ito N, et al. REM sleep is impaired by a small amount of alcohol in young women sensitive to alcohol. *Intern Med.* 2004; 43(8):679–684.

34. Answer: A

EDUCATIONAL OBJECTIVE: Identity the various physiologic changes related to sleep and sleep disorders during pregnancy.

EXPLANATION: Pregnancy leads to several hormonal and physiologic changes that might impact the development of obstructive sleep apnea (OSA). Elevated levels of estrogen during pregnancy contribute to mucosal edema and hyperemia, which increase the risk of upper airway resistance syndrome. Snoring is increased during pregnancy and decreases after delivery. The prevalence of OSA is also increased in pregnant women. Women with excessive weight gain, snoring, or excessive daytime somnolence during pregnancy should undergo polysomnography to evaluate for OSA. Clinical studies support the routine use of nasal continuous positive airway pressure (CPAP) to treat OSA during pregnancy. CPAP settings may need to be increased during later stages of pregnancy because of increased upper airway resistance and/or nasal congestion.

35. Answer: D

EDUCATIONAL OBJECTIVE: Recognize the effects of acute cocaine ingestion on sleep architecture.

EXPLANATION: Cocaine is a stimulant that increases sleep onset latency and REM latency, reduces total sleep time, and suppresses REM sleep during acute administration. REM sleep rebound is often noted after cocaine abstinence.

Reference:

Schierenbeck T, Riemann D, Berger M, et al. Effect of illicit recreational drugs upon sleep: cocaine, ecstasy and marijuana. *Sleep Med Rev.* 2008; 12(5):381–389.

36. Answer: C

EDUCATIONAL OBJECTIVE: Differentiate benzodiazepine receptor agonists from non-benzodiazepine benzodiazepine receptor agonists.

EXPLANATION: Benzodiazepine medications include temazepam, estazolam, flurazepam, and triazolam among others. They bind nonselectively to the various subunits of the gamma aminobutyric acid (GABA)-A receptor in the brain. GABA-A is a major central nervous system (CNS) inhibitory neurotransmitter. This nonselective binding is responsible not only for the hypnotic effect of benzodiazepines but also for their various side effects, such as daytime sedation, cognitive impairment, anterograde amnesia, muscle relaxation, dependency, withdrawal symptoms, and rebound insomnia on discontinuation. These medications also decrease delta sleep. In contrast, the newer non-benzodiazepine benzodiazepine receptor agonists (e.g., eszopiclone, zaleplon, and zolpidem) bind selectively to the alpha-1 subunit of the GABA-A receptor. As a result, the safety profile of these latter medications is improved with fewer side effects and a lower risk of dependency, abuse, and rebound insomnia. The hypnotic effect is comparable to that of the traditional benzodiazepines.

Reference:

Wagner J, Wagner ML. Non-benzodiazepines for the treatment of insomnia. *Sleep Med Rev.* 2000; 4(6):551–581.

37. Answer: B

EDUCATIONAL OBJECTIVE: Recognize the various effects of medications on sleep.

EXPLANATION: Medications that are alerting and can cause insomnia include the anticholinergics, antihypertensives (propanolol, atenolol, pindolol, methyldopa, and reserpine), central nervous system (CNS) stimulants (amphetamines and methylphenidate), hormones (steroids and thyroid preparations), antiparkinsonian agents (selegiline and amantadine), bronchodilators (theophylline and albuterol), and decongestants (pseudoephedrine). Lipophilic beta-blockers (propanolol) tend to disrupt sleep more than the hydrophilic beta-blockers (atenolol, sotalol, and nadolol). Withdrawal from barbiturates, benzodiazepines, sedating antidepressants, and ethanol can also lead to insomnia.

38. Answer: D

EDUCATIONAL OBJECTIVE: Recognize the different medications that can cause sedation.

EXPLANATION: The blockade of central H-1 histaminergic, alpha-1 adrenergic, and muscarinic receptors as well as the activation of gamma aminobutyric acid (GABA) receptors in the brain can give rise to sedation.

The use of tricyclic antidepressants (TCAs) has been associated with sedation. The sedating effect of tertiary amines (imipramine and trimipramine) is more pronounced compared to secondary amines (desipramine, nortriptyline, and protriptyline). TCAs inhibit serotonin and norepinephrine reuptake and block histamine-1, alpha-1 adrenergic, and cholinergic receptors. Clomipramine is the least sedating of the TCAs. Trimipramine is the only TCA that does not alter REM sleep. Selective serotonin reuptake inhibitors (SSRIs) can have various effects on sleep. Fluvoxamine and paroxetine are more likely to cause sedation, whereas fluoxetine is more commonly associated with dose-dependent insomnia. Citalopram also has alerting properties.

Trazodone is sedating and is often used as a hypnotic agent. Antipsychotic medications exert their sedative effects through blockade of the H-1 histaminergic receptors. Bupropion inhibits uptake of norepinephrine and dopamine and is associated with insomnia. First-generation H-1 histaminergic antagonists (diphenhydramine and hydroxyzine) are very lipophilic, cross the blood–brain barrier readily, and can give rise to sedation, whereas second-generation histaminergic H-1 antagonists (loratidine, terfenadine, and cetirizine) are more hydrophilic and usually do not cause sedation. Alpha-2 agonists, such as methyldopa and clonidine, produce sedation in most patients.

Most of the antiepileptic agents are sedating, especially phenobarbital; however, felbamate has been associated with both insomnia and sedation. Modafinil is a wake-promoting agent indicated in the treatment of narcolepsy.

39. Answer: A

EDUCATION OBJECTIVE: Recognize the sleep disturbances associated with the various neurologic conditions.

EXPLANATION: Various neurologic conditions are associated with insomnia, namely Parkinson disease and other movement disorders, epilepsy, dementia, and headache syndromes. Insomnia can be a direct consequence of the disease itself but also of the medications used for the disorder. Patients with Parkinson disease have insomnia with increased sleep latency and increased number of awakenings compared to normal individuals. Maintenance insomnia is more common and may be due to pain, tremor, muscle rigidity, or associated sleep disorders, such as restless legs syndrome, periodic leg movement disorders, REM sleep behavior disorder, or sleep-disordered breathing. The degree of insomnia tends to correlate with the severity of the disease. Medications used to treat Parkinson disease such as antidepressants, dopamine agonists, and anticholinergic agents can also contribute to insomnia.

Various dementing illnesses can cause sleep disruption; these include Alzheimer disease, progressive supranuclear palsy, Huntington disease, and Creutzfeldt–Jakob disease. Sleep disturbance can affect up to one third of patients with Alzheimer disease and consists of sleep disruption with loss of stage N3 and REM sleep. Nocturnal confusional arousals can occur. REM sleep behavior disorder is also more common in Alzheimer disease. Alteration in the suprachiasmatic nucleus has been implicated in the genesis of patients' disrupted circadian rhythms. Recurrent seizures during sleep can lead to sleep disruption. Initiation and maintenance insomnia are common among patients with multiple sclerosis, and pain, muscle spasms, and restless legs syndrome can all play a role in the maintenance insomnia seen in these patients.

Reference:

Dauvilliers Y. Insomnia in patients with neurodegenerative conditions. *Sleep Med.* 2007; 8(suppl 4):S27–S34.

40. Answer: B

EDUCATIONAL OBJECTIVE: Recognize the hormonal and metabolic consequences of acute sleep deprivation.

EXPLANATION: During normal sleep, release of cortisol and thyroid-stimulating hormone (TSH) is inhibited, whereas secretion of growth hormone is increased. Leptin is a hormone secreted by fat cells signaling satiety to the brain. Leptin levels are lower and are correlated to the duration of sleep deprivation. Sleep restriction also gives rise to insulin resistance with decreased rate of glucose clearance. Evening cortisol levels are increased. Finally, sleep restriction is associated with increased levels of ghrelin, a peptide released by the stomach, which increases appetite. Sleep-deprived individuals often exhibit increased hunger with craving for food rich in carbohydrate content. Increased cortisol concentrations might also contribute to the sensation of hunger.

References:

1. Spiegel K, Tasali E, Penev P, et al. Brief communication: sleep curtailment in healthy young men is associated with decreased leptin levels, elevated ghrelin levels, and increased hunger and appetite. *Ann Intern Med.* 2004; 141:846–850.
2. Spiegel K, Leproult R, Van Cauter E. Impact of sleep debt on metabolic and endocrine function. *Lancet.* 1999; 354:1435–1439.

41. Answer: D

EDUCATIONAL OBJECTIVE: Recognize the differences between tonic and phasic REM sleep.

EXPLANATION: In the awake state, there is a balance between sympathetic and parasympathetic tone. During NREM sleep, the balance tips in favor of parasympathetic activity, giving rise to a slight decrease in heart rate. During tonic REM sleep, the decrease in sympathetic activity (compared to NREM sleep) allows for a relative increase in the parasympathetic tone. Phasic REM sleep is characterized by a simultaneous increase in the sympathetic and parasympathetic activity. Great variability in heart rate and blood pressure develops during phasic REM sleep. The sudden burst of sympathetic activity during phasic REM sleep can precipitate cardiac and cerebral ischemic events.

42. Answer: A

EDUCATIONAL OBJECTIVE: Recognize the causes of 60-Hz artifact and their appropriate corrective measures.

EXPLANATION: Various appliances have a 60-Hz current activity. Differential amplifiers will record physiologic signals by increasing the difference in voltage between two electrodes while suppressing the common 60-cycle signal. Unequal impedances of the two electrodes, high electrode impedances, or lead failure will lead to increased 60-Hz activity. The electrode impedances should be low, ideally below 5,000 ohms and equal before beginning a recording. A 60-Hz artifact can be recognized by an increased amplitude of the background activity with oscillations at 60 cycles per second. The computer page can be adjusted to a 10-second page allowing easier recognition of the 60-Hz sinusoidal activity. A 60-Hz filter can also be used to decrease the interference as a last resort.

43. Answer: C

EDUCATIONAL OBJECTIVE: Identify the causes of continuous positive airway pressure (CPAP) nonadherence.

EXPLANATION: Patients often overestimate the number of hours of CPAP use. Only about 40% to 60% of patients use CPAP 4 to 6 hours each night. Many CPAP machines have a Smart Card from which compliance data can be downloaded. Serial phone discussions have been shown to improve CPAP compliance when done at the initiation of treatment. Intensive education about obstructive sleep apnea and its cardiovascular consequences should be done. A systematic approach is necessary to determine whether the patient has some mask problems, nasal symptoms, claustrophobia, or pressure intolerance. Discomfort with the mask is a very common complaint. Air leaks can manifest as a dry mouth sensation in the morning. A chinstrap should be added if the patient suffers from mouth leaks; a full face mask is another possible approach. Nasal obstruction can be alleviated by saline nasal spray, nasal steroids, heated humidification, or the use of a full face mask. Heated humidification has been shown to improve CPAP compliance. If the patient experiences trouble exhaling against the CPAP pressure or develops aerophagia, an expiratory pressure release (EPR) mechanism maybe added to the CPAP device. Bi-level positive airway pressure is another alternative to address the problem of aerophagia. Nasal pillows may be employed to counter claustrophobia.

References:

1. Aloia MS, Stanchina M, Arnedt JT, et al. Treatment adherence and outcomes in flexible vs standard continuous positive airway pressure therapy. *Chest.* 2005; 127:2085–2093.
2. Massie CA, Hart RW, Peralez K, et al. Effects of humidification on nasal symptoms and compliance in sleep apnea patients using continuous positive airway pressure. *Chest.* 1999; 116(2):403–408.

44. Answer: A

EDUCATIONAL OBJECTIVE: Recognize potential cardiovascular consequences of untreated obstructive sleep apnea (OSA).

EXPLANATION: Cardiac output is decreased during an apneic episode because of decreased preload and increased afterload. Increase in blood pressure and heart rate occurs at the termination of the apneic episode. Repetitive arousals and hypoxia lead to increased activity of the sympathetic nervous system, which is maintained even during the daytime and manifests as hypertension. Epidemiologic studies have established a strong relationship between OSA and systemic hypertension. The absence of a physiologic nocturnal dip in blood pressure among patients with OSA is predictive of adverse cardiovascular events. Increased levels of fibrinogen, evidence of a hypercoagulability state as well as platelet activation are present in patients with OSA. OSA increases the risk of stroke even after adjusting for confounding factors. Patients with OSA also are more likely to develop coronary artery disease. Cardiac arrhythmias such as brady-tachycardia, brady-arrhythmia, and atrial fibrillation are more common with OSA patients. Hypoxia during the apneic episode contributes to bradycardia through vagal nerve stimulation, whereas reflex tachycardia occurs with apnea termination. Untreated OSA patients are more likely to have recurrent atrial fibrillation after cardioversion compared to normal subjects without OSA.

References:

1. Yaggi HK, Concato J, Kernan WN, et al. Obstructive sleep apnea as a risk factor for stroke and death. *N Engl J Med.* 2005; 353:2034–2041.
2. Peppard PE, Young T, Palta M, et al. Prospective study of the association between sleep-disordered breathing and hypertension. *N Engl J Med.* 2000; 342:1378–1384.
3. Kanagala R, Murali NS, Friedman PA, et al. Obstructive sleep apnea and the recurrence of atrial fibrillation. *Circulation.* 2003; 107:2589–2594.

45. Answer: B

EDUCATIONAL OBJECTIVE: Recognize the electroencephalographic (EEG) and clinical features of alpha intrusion.

EXPLANATION: Alpha EEG wave intrusion can be present during all stages of NREM sleep and renders the scoring of sleep stages more challenging. It consists of brief repetitive superimposition of alpha waves on the background EEG tracing in various sleep stages during NREM sleep. It is associated with certain clinical conditions that will disrupt sleep such as fibromyalgia, chronic pain syndrome, and depression and is felt to be an indication of nonrestorative sleep. Nonetheless, it is neither specific nor sensitive for any disorder and can be encountered in normal healthy individuals as well.

46. Answer: D

EDUCATIONAL OBJECTIVE: Recognize the effect of medications on the electroencephalogram.

EXPLANATION: Benzodiazepines may produce pseudo-spindles on the electroencephalogram. Pseudo-spindles have a higher frequency at 15 to 16 Hz than regular spindles which have frequencies of 12 to 14 Hz. Sleep spindles originate in the central vertex region, occur in small bursts, and last from 0.5 to 3 seconds. They are typically present during stage N2 sleep. Pseudo-spindles may also appear during REM sleep.

47. Answer: C

EDUCATIONAL OBJECTIVE: Adequately interpret multiple sleep latency test (MSLT) results on the basis of the appropriate clinical context.

EXPLANATION: This patient suffers from delayed sleep phase syndrome. He had no symptoms of excessive daytime somnolence until he started his new job that requires an early wake time. A careful sleep history, sleep diary for 2 weeks, and a polysomnography preceding the MSLT are necessary to ensure an adequate sleep time to correctly interpret the MSLT results. The finding of two sleep-onset REM periods is suggestive of narcolepsy if associated with a short mean sleep latency but is not specific for this disorder. Sleep deprivation, delayed sleep phase syndrome, abrupt withdrawal of REM suppressant medications, depression, acute cocaine withdrawal, and obstructive sleep apnea can be associated with the presence of REM sleep during the MSLT. Sleep-disordered breathing or movement disorders should be adequately treated before undergoing an MSLT if narcolepsy is suspected. Conversely, REM latency can be increased and REM sleep duration suppressed if the patient is taking REM suppressant medications or stimulants; these medications should be withdrawn for at least 2 weeks before performing an MSLT.

48. Answer: C

EDUCATIONAL OBJECTIVE: Understand the significance of a blunted heart rate variability in patients with obstructive sleep apnea (OSA).

EXPLANATION: Patients with OSA have an increased risk of adverse cardiovascular events. Heart rate variability is a noninvasive way of assessing the response of the cardiac autonomic nervous system. During an apneic episode, there is an increased sympathetic nervous system activity, activation of the renin–angiotensin–aldosterone system, and a surge in blood pressure. The heart rate variability is decreased among patients with OSA, is correlated to the severity of the disease, and portends a worse cardiovascular outcome.

49. Answer: B

EDUCATIONAL OBJECTIVE: Describe the effects of antidepressant agents on sleep.

EXPLANATION: In addition to inhibiting serotonin reuptake, fluoxetine and paroxetine also block norepinephrine reuptake. Paroxetine is among the most sedating of the selective serotonin reuptake inhibitors (SSRIs). SSRIs tend to decrease total sleep time as well as REM sleep and are more commonly linked to complaints of insomnia.

50. Answer: D

EDUCATIONAL OBJECTIVE: Recognize the symptoms of rebound insomnia.

EXPLANATION: This patient was instructed to abruptly discontinue her benzodiazepine agent that led to rebound insomnia. Rebound insomnia is characterized by sudden exacerbation of insomnia compared to baseline levels after discontinuation of benzodiazepine use. Benzodiazepine withdrawal manifests as worsening insomnia with anxiety, tremor, irritability, and, in rare instances, seizures. This is more commonly seen with shorter-acting benzodiazepines. Benzodiazepines bind nonselectively to the gamma aminobutyric acid (GABA) receptor complex, which mediates muscle relaxation, antianxiety, hypnotic effect, and antiseizure activity. Benzodiazepine use should be tapered slowly to avoid rebound insomnia or withdrawal symptoms. In contrast, the newer hypnotic agents, such as zaleplon, eszopiclone or zolpidem, are less likely to cause rebound insomnia or major withdrawal symptoms when stopped abruptly.

Reference:

Wagner J, Wagner ML. Non-benzodiazepines for the treatment of insomnia. *Sleep Med Rev.* 2000; 4(6):551–581.

51. Answer: D

EDUCATIONAL OBJECTIVE: Describe the clinical features and management of bruxism.

EXPLANATION: Bruxism is a common parasomnia characterized by crunching and grinding of the teeth at night. Bruxers are most often not aware of the parasomnia, but may complain of temporomandibular joint (TMJ) or jaw discomfort in the morning, or occasionally headaches. Bed partners can be disturbed by the sound generated by bruxism. Dental examination may reveal abnormal tooth wear and damage. It can occur during any stage of sleep, but is more frequent during stage N2 sleep. Polysomnography demonstrates a sudden increased electromyographic (EMG), electroencephalographic (EEG), and electrooculographic (EOG) tone with muscle activity occurring in a rhythmic pattern. Seizures can mimic bruxism and should be excluded. Alcohol intake and certain medications, such as amphetamines or selective serotonin reuptake inhibitors, can worsen bruxism. A mouth guard should be worn at night to prevent tooth wear. Malocclusion, if present, should be corrected. Relaxation is a useful adjunctive therapeutic strategy since bruxism may be aggravated by stress.

52. Answer: C

EDUCATIONAL OBJECTIVE: Discuss the clinical features and management of REM sleep behavior disorder (RBD).

EXPLANATION: This scenario is typical of RBD. The wife reports violent motor behavior occurring during sleep, particularly at the end of the night when percentage of REM sleep is greater. Patients do not generally report excessive daytime somnolence despite sleep disruption due to violent behavior. Most often the patient is brought by the bed partner with some type of injury to either one or both. Patients can recall their dreams, which are commonly action-filled or violent in nature. RBD affects mostly older men with a higher incidence after age 50 years. Acute RBD can develop following use of certain medications, such as monoamine oxidase inhibitors (MAOIs), tricyclic antidepressants (TCAs), venlafaxine, and selective serotonin reuptake inhibitors (SSRIs). Most cases are idiopathic but RBD can also herald specific neurologic disorders, such as Parkinson disease, neurodegenerative disorder, dementia, or multiple sclerosis, with normal pressure hydrocephalus, cerebrovascular accident, or subarachnoid hemorrhage. A thorough neurologic examination should be performed.

RBD is due to a loss of atonia during REM sleep, thus allowing some complex motor activities to emerge during this stage of sleep. Experimental bilateral lesions of the peri-locus coeruleus in cats have reproduced RBD features. Polysomnography demonstrates increased electromyographic (EMG) tone during REM sleep associated with complex motor behavior. Clonazepam is very effective in treating RBD. Melatonin is another possible therapeutic option. Safety measures should be emphasized to prevent injury to patients and their bed partners.

Patients with posttraumatic stress disorder (PTSD) have terrible nightmares but do not exhibit aggressive complex motor activity. Sleep terrors are more common in young children and there is often poor or no dream recall.

Reference:

Gagnon J-F, Postuma R, Montplaisr J. Update on the pharmacology of REM sleep behavior disorder. *Neurology.* 2006; 67:742–747.

53. Answer: C

EDUCATIONAL OBJECTIVE: Identify the characteristics of rhythmic movement disorders such as body rocking.

EXPLANATION: Body rocking is a form of rhythmic movement disorder that also includes head rolling and head banging. Compared with the latter, body rocking affects younger children with greatest prevalence at 9 to12 months. It is also described in children with mental retardation or autism. These disorders rarely persist into adulthood. Etiology is unclear. Repetitive movements of the head and neck occur during drowsiness and can persist into all stages of sleep. Duration is usually less than 15 minutes. Body rocking is usually considered a benign condition. Protective measures are recommended. Rarely, benzodiazepines may be necessary to prevent injury.

54. Answer: B

EDUCATIONAL OBJECTIVE: Recognize the characteristics of sleepwalking.

EXPLANATION: Sleepwalking is more common in children than in adults and peaks around 4 to 8 years old, but can persist into adulthood. It is typically seen during the first third of the night and is a disorder of arousal usually arising from stage N3 sleep. The patient commonly has total amnesia of the event and, if awakened during sleepwalking, appears confused. Sleepwalking can be precipitated by fever, sleep deprivation, and medications, such as tricyclic antidepressants (TCA) and lithium. Safety measures as well as the avoidance of triggering factors should be emphasized. Benzodiazepines might be helpful in severe cases.

55. Answer: C

EDUCATIONAL OBJECTIVE: Identify conditions associated with periodic leg movements.

EXPLANATION: The prevalence of periodic leg movement disorder (PLMD) increases with age, most commonly affecting patients older than 60 years of age. It can be associated with restless legs syndrome, REM sleep behavior disorder, narcolepsy, and obstructive sleep apnea. Periodic leg movements occur during sleep approximately every 5 to 90 seconds and last 0.5 to 5 seconds. They can occasionally cause arousals, but patients are generally unaware of the movements. Among adults, a periodic leg movement index above 15 per hour is considered abnormal in the appropriate clinical setting. It might also be an incidental finding during polysomnography in an otherwise asymptomatic period, in which case, it likely does not warrant treatment. Symptomatic patients may benefit from a dopaminergic agonist taken prior to bedtime. Iron deficiency (i.e., low serum ferritin levels), if present, should also be corrected.

56. Answer: A and B

EDUCATIONAL OBJECTIVE: Recognize the sleep–wake disturbances caused by traumatic brain injury (TBI).

EXPLANATION: Studies reveal that new onset of sleep–wake disturbances is very common after TBI, affecting up to 72% of patients. The most common complaints are excessive daytime somnolence, fatigue, posttraumatic hypersomnia (increase in total sleep time of about 2 hours compared to baseline levels). Insomnia is seen in a minority of patients and is more likely related to nocturnal pain. Objective hypersomnia documented by shortened mean sleep latency on multiple sleep latency test (MSLT) has been documented in about a quarter of patients in some studies. Another study demonstrated that cerebrospinal fluid (CSF) levels of hypocretin-1 were decreased after acute traumatic brain injury. Traumatic brain injury may possibly give rise to structural damage of the hypothalamus, including the hypocretin neurons.

Complaints of excessive daytime somnolence can persist for up to 1 year after injury.

References:

1. Castriotta RJ, Wilde MC, Lai JM, et al. Prevalence and consequences of sleep disorders in traumatic brain injury. *J Clin Sleep Med.* 2007; 3:349–356.
2. Baumann CR, Werth E, Stocker R, et al. Sleep–wake disturbances 6 months after traumatic brain injury. *Brain.* 2007; 130:1873–1883.

57. Answer: A

EDUCATIONAL OBJECTIVE: Recognize the characteristics of complex sleep apnea.

EXPLANATION: Complex sleep apnea is characterized by the development of central apneas in some obstructive sleep apnea patients when placed on continuous positive airway pressure (CPAP) therapy; thus complex sleep apnea patients have significant residual apnea–hypopnea index (AHI) due to the onset of central apneas on CPAP therapy. Patients are more frequently male but have comparable underlying cardiovascular disease than the obstructive sleep apnea patients. They have less insomnia than central sleep apnea patients. It is believed that complex sleep apnea patients are more likely to become hypocapnic during sleep, leading to the central apneic events. Adaptive servoventilation (ASV) is a new modality that targets 90% of a patient's minute ventilation while adjusting pressure support settings breath by breath. If the patient has a central apneic event, the device will deliver airflow. Conversely, no airflow will be delivered if spontaneous breathing is present, thus preventing subsequent hypocapnic episodes. ASV in several studies was found to be more effective than CPAP or bi-level positive airway pressure (BPAP) therapy in decreasing AHI and in improving sleep quality in this patient population.

References:

1. Morgenthaler TI, Kagramanov V, Hanak V, et al. Complex sleep apnea syndrome: is it a unique clinical syndrome? *Sleep.* 2006; 29(9):1203–1209.
2. Allam JS, Olson EJ, Gay PC, et al. Efficacy of adaptive servoventilation in treatment of complex and central sleep apnea syndrome. *Chest.* 2007; 132:1839–1846.

58. Answer: B

EDUCATIONAL OBJECTIVE: Enumerate the various cytokine and immunologic changes seen with sleep deprivation.

EXPLANATION: Infection stimulates the formation of proinflammatory cytokines, such as interleukin (IL-1) and tumor necrosis factor (TNF), which are somnogenic and tend to increase stage N3 sleep. Animal studies have shown that sleep deprivation alters cellular and natural immunity, thus possibly compromising host defenses. Total chronic sleep deprivation leads to bacteremia and death. Partial sleep deprivation reduces cellular immunity by decreasing natural killer function. A deficit in monocyte and T cell lymphocyte population leads to decreased production of IL-2. An increase in markers of systemic inflammation, namely, IL-1, interferon, and TNF-α, has been described during sleep deprivation. Sleep deprivation has also been found to decrease immune response to vaccination in humans. Stage N3 sleep is associated with elevated levels of IL-2 in humans.

Reference:

Irwin M. Effects of sleep and sleep loss on immunity and cytokines. *Brain Behav Immun.* 2002; 16:503–512.

59. Answer: B

EDUCATIONAL OBJECTIVE: Recognize the effect of sleep deprivation on sleep architecture.

EXPLANATION: Acute partial sleep deprivation is associated with reduction in stage N2 and REM sleep. During chronic partial sleep deprivation, stage N3 sleep is maintained but REM sleep is reduced. An equal amount of sleep is not required to recover from sleep loss. On the first recovery night, there is an increase in stage N3 sleep, whereas the second recovery night is characterized by increased REM sleep.

60. Answer: B

EDUCATIONAL OBJECTIVE: Recognize the metabolic consequences of sleep deprivation.

EXPLANATION: Epidemiologic studies in children have linked sleep deprivation with an increased future risk of obesity. The US Nurses Health Study reported a significant increased risk of diabetes in women sleeping less than 5 hours even after correcting for confounding factors. Similar findings were noted in males sleeping less than 6 hours per night in the Massachusetts Male Aging Study. A study among young healthy lean subjects revealed impaired glucose tolerance after sleep curtailment.

References:

1. Spiegel K, Leproult R, Van Cauter E. Impact of sleep debt on metabolic and endocrine function. *Lancet.* 1999; 354:1435–1439.
2. Ayas NT, White DP, Al-Delaimy WK, et al. A prospective study of self-reported sleep duration and incident diabetes in women. *Diabetes Care.* 2003; 26(2):380–384.
3. Yaggi HK, Araujo AB, McKinlay JB. Sleep duration as a risk factor for the development of type 2 diabetes. Massachusetts Male Aging Study. *Diabetes Care.* 2006; 29:657–661.

61. Answer: C

EDUCATIONAL OBJECTIVE: Describe the changes in cerebral blood flow that occur during sleep.

EXPLANATION: Cerebral blood flow is influenced by regional cerebral metabolism while awake, including changes in Po_2 and Pco_2. An increase in Pco_2 will increase cortical blood flow due to hypercapnia-induced vasodilation. During

NREM sleep, cerebral blood flow and metabolism are decreased despite a rise in Pco_2 due to a physiologic reduction in alveolar ventilation. A reduction in cerebrovascular response to hypercapnia during NREM sleep can render cerebral perfusion more vulnerable to metabolic changes. In contrast, cerebral blood flow is markedly increased during tonic REM sleep compared to wakefulness. Patients with obstructive sleep apnea have impaired cerebral autoregulation that can increase their risk of stroke.

Reference:

Meadows GE, Dunroy HM, Morrell MJ, et al. Hypercapnic cerebral vascular reactivity is decreased, in humans, during sleep compared with wakefulness. *J Appl Physiol.* 2003; 94:2197–2202.

62. Answer: B

EDUCATIONAL OBJECTIVE: Describe the appropriate management for advanced sleep phase syndrome (ASPS).

EXPLANATION: This patient suffers from ASPS, which is characterized by a bedtime that is earlier than is conventional or desired. It is seen more commonly in the elderly who might complain of an early bedtime and early rising time that interferes with normal daily activities. They may also raise concern about an early awakening and about not getting enough sleep. Nonetheless, their total sleep time and sleep quality are usually adequate. A mutation in a clock component has been demonstrated in the familial form of ASPS. A careful sleep history and a sleep diary for at least 2 weeks are of importance in establishing the diagnosis. Actigraphy can also be used to demonstrate early bedtimes and early awakenings. There is no indication for a polysomnography unless an additional sleep diagnosis is being considered. Exposure to bright light in the evening close to bedtime will result in a phase delay of the circadian sleep–wake cycle. Administration of melatonin in the morning might be theoretically beneficial but there is no convincing data showing adequate clinical efficacy. Good sleep hygiene with avoidance of naps should be emphasized. Depression in the elderly can also manifest as early morning awakenings and should be considered as a differential diagnosis.

Reference:

Toh KL, Jones CR, He Y, et al. An hPer2 phosphorylation site mutation in familial advanced sleep phase syndrome. *Science.* 2001; 291:1040–1043.

63. Answer: C

EDUCATIONAL OBJECTIVE: Describe the clinical features of the various neuromuscular disorders.

EXPLANATION: Myotonic dystrophy is a distal myopathy that can affect pharyngeal and laryngeal muscles as well as respiratory muscles including the diaphragm. During REM sleep, there is normally a physiologic muscle atonia involving the respiratory muscles with sparing of the diaphragm. In addition, hypoxic and hypercapnic ventilatory responses are decreased during sleep compared to wakefulness. Thus, alveolar hypoventilation can develop in patients with myotonic dystrophy predominantly during REM sleep because of diaphragmatic weakness. Patients also have an increased risk of obstructive and central sleep apneas. Their oropharyngeal muscles may become so weak that they are unable to effectively overcome upper airway obstruction. The sleep-related alveolar hypoventilation can be exacerbated in presence of obstructive sleep apnea and microatelectasis. The presence of significant nocturnal desaturation, especially in REM sleep, increases the risk of developing pulmonary hypertension.

64. Answer: D

EDUCATIONAL OBJECTIVE: Describe the clinical features of hypnic jerks.

EXPLANATION: Hypnic jerks or sleep starts occur in up to 70% of the population. They consist of sudden and brief contractions of the muscles of the legs or, less commonly, the arms during sleep onset. Occasionally, they can precipitate sleep initiation insomnia. Hypnic jerks can be associated with an abrupt sensation of falling or vivid dreams. Episodes can be aggravated by stress, sleep deprivation, and excessive caffeine intake. Differential diagnoses include restless legs syndrome, periodic leg movement disorder, fragmentary myoclonus, and brief epileptic myoclonus. Fragmentary myoclonus consists of small jerks that occur in a bilateral and symmetrical manner and persist into sleep. Epileptic myoclonus persists into sleep and is associated with other symptoms of seizure disorder.

65. Answer: B

EDUCATIONAL OBJECTIVE: Recognize effects of sleep deprivation on cognitive function.

EXPLANATION: Waking brain function is influenced by sleep loss with impairment of attentive skills, memory, and higher executive functions. Dynamic performance shifts occur as a result of homeostatic and circadian drives. Cognitive performance reaches a nadir in the mid-afternoon after peaking in mid-morning for individuals with typical sleep–wake patterns.

Specific cognitive performance degradations include behavioral lapses, errors of commission, and response slowing. Wake state instability leads to variable cognitive performance. Executive functions that are impaired include creative thinking, fluency, and nonverbal planning. Increased time-on-task is associated with a progressive worsening of performance.

66. Answer: D

EDUCATIONAL OBJECTIVE: Recognize cardiac rhythm changes with sleep.

EXPLANATION: Electrocardiographic monitoring performed during polysomnography may reveal a variety of findings of potential significance. Many patients have no previous electrocardiographic assessments. Premature beats and intermittent bundle-branch block may occur during sleep without obvious precipitating respiratory events. Paroxysmal atrial fibrillation may occur from increased vagal activity. Patients with obstructive sleep apnea often demonstrate "brady-tachycardia" with heart rate slowing during the onset of an apnea followed by a marked increased heart rate in the postapneic period.

In general, heart rate slows during NREM sleep due to increased parasympathetic activity. Sinus pauses during sleep may occur in healthy individuals, particularly during tonic REM sleep, secondary to the effects of further increased parasympathetic tone on atrioventricular node conduction.

67. Answer: D

EDUCATIONAL OBJECTIVE: Recognize potential uses of actigraphy.

EXPLANATION: Actigraphs are small devices that record and store data related to movement. They may be worn like a wristwatch and data can be recorded continuously over an extended period of time. An interface with a computer allows graphic correlation of activity with algorithmic estimates of sleep or wakefulness based on patient movements.

The accuracy of sleep–wake estimates may vary with different devices and are less accurate in patients with insomnia or movement disorders. Nevertheless, actigraphy may prove useful in assessment of patients with insomnia, somnolence, or suspected circadian rhythm disorders. Actigraphs may also be helpful in evaluating response to behavioral and treatment interventions.

68. Answer: A

EDUCATIONAL OBJECTIVE: Recognize "false-negative" oximetry in the assessment of sleep-disordered breathing.

EXPLANATION: Overnight oximetry is often performed as a screening tool for sleep apnea. Abnormal oximetry may reveal evidence of possible sleep apnea, sleep-related hypoventilation, or chronic hypoxemia.

A "normal" oximetry does not exclude significant sleep apnea. Patients with normal baseline oxygen saturation may have frequent but brief apneas–hypopneas that do not result in obvious or prolonged oxygen desaturations. Occasionally, oximetry tracings may reveal a sawtooth pattern resulting from repetitive subtle desaturations.

69. Answer: D

EDUCATIONAL OBJECTIVE: Understand the use of subjective tests of sleepiness.

EXPLANATION: The Epworth Sleepiness Scale (ESS) is a self-rated scale based on patient responses to the likelihood of falling asleep during eight situations over time. Ratings of 0 to 3 are reported for each question and a score between 0 and 24 is generated, with higher scores correlating with increased sleepiness.

Scores of 10 or higher suggest significant sleepiness but do not provide specific causes or diagnoses. ESS scores do not correlate with multiple sleep latency test (MSLT) data.

70. Answer: C

EDUCATIONAL OBJECTIVE: Recognize polysomnographic patterns of the wake stage.

EXPLANATION: The awake electroencephalography (EEG) is characterized primarily by alpha activity with a frequency of 8 to 12 Hz in adults. Additional waveforms may also be seen, including beta activity (18 to 35 Hz) seen with drowsiness or with sedating medications and lambda waves seen in the posterior leads during reading.

Alpha activity is reduced with sleep onset but is also significantly suppressed by eye openings while awake. This is often most evident in the occipital leads. Electrooculographic patterns with eyes-open wakefulness include eye blinks and rapid eye movements. With eye closure, alpha activity increases and slow rolling eye movements may develop.

71. Answer: B

EDUCATIONAL OBJECTIVE: Familiarity with epidemiology, pathophysiology, and therapy of sleep bruxism.

EXPLANATION: Sleep bruxism is a parasomnia characterized by repetitive grinding and clenching of the teeth. It is more common in children than in adults with approximately 5% to 8% of adults reporting symptoms. It may be diagnosed by noting significant wear on dentition. It is a significant cause of dental/jaw pain and temporomandibular disorder (TMD).

Polysomnographic (PSG) findings demonstrate rhythmic jaw electromyographic (EMG) discharges exceeding 25% of maximal clench when awake. Three types of episodes are identified: tonic activity of greater than 2 seconds, phasic activity lasting between 0.25 and 2 seconds, and mixed activity. Episodes are separated by at least 3 seconds. They occur more commonly in stages N1 and N2 sleep than during REM sleep.

No specific treatment has been established by controlled trials. Oral devices may protect dentition and alleviate pain. Benzodiazepines have been reported to reduce bruxing motor activity. Selective serotonin reuptake inhibitors (SSRIs) have no effect on bruxism and are associated with grinding and daytime clenching.

72. Answer: B

EDUCATIONAL OBJECTIVE: Understand the pathophysiology of sleep-disordered breathing in congestive heart failure.

EXPLANATION: Central sleep apnea is often seen in patients with congestive heart failure with a pattern of periodic breathing or Cheyne–Stokes respiration (CSR). This is a consequence of increased circulatory time secondary to left ventricular dysfunction or valvular dysfunction. This is especially common in cases of atrial fibrillation. Patients have an increased respiratory drive from pulmonary congestion which, in turn, gives rise to hypocapnea. The decreased loop gain results in a recurrent pattern of central apneas as CO_2 levels fall below the apneic threshold followed by a hyperpneic ventilatory response. Arousals coincide with the peak of hyperpnea.

Therapeutic options for this respiratory disturbance include maximizing cardiac function with diuretics, beta-blockers, and afterload-reducing agents. Additional interventions may include nocturnal oxygen, positive airway pressure therapy, or adaptive servoventilation.

73. Answer: D

EDUCATIONAL OBJECTIVE: Recognize the significance of obstructive sleep apnea in patients with comorbid pulmonary disease.

EXPLANATION: Overlap syndrome is defined by the occurrence of obstructive sleep apnea (OSA) in patients with intrinsic pulmonary disease, most typically obstructive lung disease. As chronic obstructive pulmonary disease (COPD) and OSA are common, the overlap syndrome is commonly encountered.

Patients with overlap syndrome display disproportionately worse hypercapnia and nocturnal oxygen desaturation than expected based on the severity of obstructive lung disease. It should be suspected in patients with mild to moderate pulmonary obstruction who present with hypercapnia. These patients have an increased risk of developing hypercapnic respiratory failure and pulmonary hypertension compared to patients with OSA alone. Ideally, therapy should address both obstructive lung disease and OSA. Continuous positive airway pressure support should be utilized and nocturnal oxygen therapy may be required for refractory hypoxemia. Bi-level positive airway pressure support may potentially be of benefit; however, unlike obesity hypoventilation syndrome, no definitive data exist for its use in overlap syndrome.

Reference:

Weitzenblam E, Chaouat A, Kessler R, et al. Overlap syndrome: obstructive sleep apnea in patients with chronic obstructive lung disease. *Proc Am Thorac Soc.* 2008; 5:237–241.

74. Answer: C

EDUCATIONAL OBJECTIVE: Understand the clinical features of upper airway resistance syndrome (UARS).

EXPLANATION: Many consider UARS as a form of mild sleep-disordered breathing characterized by recurrent subtle respiratory effort–related arousals (RERAs). These events do not meet the criteria for apneas or hypopneas and are usually detectable only by nasal or esophageal pressure monitoring. Accordingly, patients with UARS will demonstrate a normal apnea–hypopnea index (AHI) without evidence of significant nocturnal oxygen desaturations. By definition, these patients have daytime symptoms secondary to the repeated arousals and the resulting sleep fragmentation. Treatment options include continuous positive airway pressure (CPAP) as well as more conservative approaches including weight loss and treatment of reversible nasal obstruction.

75. Answer: C

EDUCATIONAL OBJECTIVE: Understand the role of oral appliances in the treatment of obstructive sleep apnea (OSA).

EXPLANATION: Oral appliances may be effective for mild to moderate OSA. They might also significantly reduce the severity of more severe OSA. The mechanism of action involves moving the base of the tongue forward as the mandible is stabilized to the maxilla by the device. Tongue-retaining devices have been described but are rarely utilized currently.

A trained dental specialist should be involved in fashioning an appropriate device to reduce potential oral and temporomandibular joint (TMJ) complications. Appliances do not benefit patients with central apneas or hypoventilation and may not be effective for patients with OSA who have significant oxygen desaturation.

References:

1. Kushida CA, Morgenthaler TI, Littner MR, et al. Practice parameters for the treatment of snoring and obstructive sleep apnea with oral appliances: an update for 2005. *Sleep.* 2006; 29:240–243.
2. Chan ASL, Lee RWW, Cistulli PA. Dental appliance treatment for obstructive sleep apnea. *Chest.* 2007; 132:693–699.

76. Answer: D

EDUCATIONAL OBJECTIVE: Recognize the importance of perioperative management of patients with obstructive sleep apnea (OSA).

EXPLANATION: Preoperative protocols should identify patients at risk for OSA as well as those with a known diagnosis of OSA. Assessments should include a detailed history with specific questions about symptoms suggestive of OSA and examination to assess potential airway issues. Elective surgery may potentially be delayed until polysomnography is performed and appropriate therapy is instituted.

Intraoperative management should recognize the increased risks for upper airway collapse and respiratory suppression. Medication selection should consider the potential for adverse postoperative effects. Local anesthesia should be used whenever possible. If moderate sedation is utilized, continuous monitoring with both oximetry and capnography is advised. If general anesthesia is utilized, a secure airway is preferred.

Extubation should be delayed until patients are alert enough to protect their airways and maintain respiratory drive. It should be performed whenever possible in a nonsupine position. Supplemental oxygen is recommended for patients with OSA until they are able to maintain adequate saturations. Continuous positive airway pressure (CPAP) or noninvasive ventilatory support may be needed in some patients in the immediately postoperative period. Regional analgesia should also be considered to reduce the need for systemic opioids for pain control.

77. Answer: C

EDUCATIONAL OBJECTIVE: Recognize stage N2 sleep electroencephalography (EEG) morphology.

EXPLANATION: NREM stage N2 sleep is defined by the appearance of either sleep spindles or K-complexes. In addition, N2 sleep has delta activity occupying <20% of the epoch. This stage of sleep comprises more than half of the total sleep time in most individuals.

Sleep spindles are bursts of 12- to 14-Hz activity with a characteristic shape and duration of 0.5 to 2 seconds. They represent oscillations of the reticular nucleus of the thalamus. They may persist into stage N3 sleep.

K-complexes are large-amplitude biphasic deflections of greater than 0.5 seconds, which occur at a frequency of 1 to 3 per minute. An initial sharp negative voltage deflection is followed by a slow positive tracing. K-complexes represent cortical slow-wave activity.

78. Answer: D

EDUCATIONAL OBJECTIVE: Recognize the significance of REM-related apnea in symptomatic patients with a normal apnea–hypopnea index (AHI).

EXPLANATION: The frequency of apneas and hypopneas and the severity of oxygen desaturation typically increase during REM sleep. Some patients will demonstrate significant apnea exclusively during REM sleep. This pattern may be more frequent in females with obstructive sleep apnea.

Various factors may contribute to the emergence of increased obstructive respiratory events during REM sleep. REM sleep respiration, compared with NREM sleep, is more unstable with an increased respiratory rate and reduced tidal volume. During REM sleep there is a reduction in muscle tone of the upper airway, impairment of genioglossus reflexes to increased negative pressure and reduced chemosensitivity to O_2 and CO_2. Interestingly, critical closing pressures (P_{crit}) do not appear to be significantly different in REM compared to NREM sleep.

Therapy should be started for symptomatic patients with REM-related apnea. Continuous positive airway pressure (CPAP) or oral appliances may be considered, and their effectiveness should be confirmed by follow-up sleep studies. The use of auto-titrating PAP has been advocated for patients with REM-related apnea and in patients with disparately higher pressure requirements for REM sleep. Nasal oxygen alone is unlikely to be of significant benefit.

79. Answer: C

EDUCATIONAL OBJECTIVE: Recognize anatomic considerations of the upper airway in obstructive sleep apnea (OSA).

EXPLANATION: Anatomic variations of the upper airway contribute to the pathophysiology of OSA. Abnormalities of both soft tissue and bony structures should be considered in the evaluation of OSA and may direct specific therapies for the disorder.

Recognized anatomic patterns associated with increased risk for apnea include a high-arched palate, hypoplastic mandible, retropositioning of the hyoid and maxilla, more elliptical airway, increased tongue volume, elongated and thickened soft palate, and enlarged parapharyngeal fat pads. These factors are likely responsible for familial and ethnic tendencies for OSA. Nasal obstruction may also contribute to severity of the disorder.

The importance of anatomic factors should always be considered in the treatment of sleep-disordered breathing, particularly when evaluating patients with severe disease or when considering alternative therapies. Nasal obstruction, if present, should be treated aggressively. Various airway imaging modalities may be pursued including cephalometric analysis with computed tomography (CT) or magnetic resonance imaging (MRI). A direct visualization using nasopharyngoscopy with the patient performing the Müller maneuver may also prove helpful. These assessments may better identify patients most likely to benefit from oral appliances or uvulopalatopharyngoplasty. Advanced surgical procedures, such as genioglossus advancement, hyoid myotomy, laser midline glossectomy, and lingualplasty, may also be considered for severe disease but should be performed only by experienced maxillofacial surgeons.

80. Answer: C

EDUCATIONAL OBJECTIVE: Recognize the significance of mild sleep-disordered breathing.

EXPLANATION: On the basis of the American Academy of Sleep Medicine (AASM) Practice Parameter guidelines, continuous positive airway pressure (CPAP) therapy is indicated for an apnea–hypopnea index (AHI) of 15 or higher. For mild obstructive apnea with an AHI of 5 to 14, CPAP is not indicated in the absence of documented symptoms of excessive daytime sleepiness, impaired cognition, mood disorders or insomnia, or documented hypertension, ischemic heart disease or a history of stroke. This patient has no specific symptoms or medical conditions to justify the use of CPAP.

While data confirms the efficacy of oral appliances for mild to moderate OSA, there is no convincing evidence to definitively support the role of airway surgery for OSA. Conservative management with lifestyle changes may correct mild OSA. Follow-up is warranted since OSA may worsen over time, and even mild OSA (AHI 5 to 15) is associated with an odds ratio of 2.03 for developing systemic hypertension over the subsequent 4 years.

Reference:

Kushida CA, Littner MR, Hirshkowitz M, et al. Practice parameters for the use of continuous and bi-level positive airway pressure devices to treat adult patients with sleep-related breathing disorders. *Sleep*. 2006; 29(3):375–380.

81. Answer: C

EDUCATIONAL OBJECTIVE: Understand the role of obesity and weight loss in obstructive sleep apnea (OSA).

EXPLANATION: Obesity is a reversible risk factor for the development of OSA. Nonetheless, up to a third of patients with OSA may be nonobese. Obesity is associated with increased fat deposition in the lateral pharyngeal walls with subsequent reduction in the caliber and shape of the upper airway. In addition, more significant obesity may alter pulmonary mechanics by reducing supine lung volumes and further increasing the likelihood of airway instability.

Modest weight loss of 10% of body weight may reduce the severity of OSA and potentially normalize apnea–hypopnea index (AHI) in some, but not all, patients with mild OSA. Weight loss may also result in a reduction in positive airway pressure (PAP) requirements. Bariatric surgery should be considered in morbidly obese patients with severe OSA, especially if PAP therapy is ineffective or poorly tolerated. Just as weight loss may lessen OSA, weight gain may be associated with increased severity of OSA and increased therapeutic PAP requirements.

82. Answer: D

EDUCATIONAL OBJECTIVE: Identify the medications that can affect slow-wave sleep (SWS).

EXPLANATION: Although the concept of utilizing pharmacologic agents to increase the percentage of SWS has been proposed by some investigators and while some medications appear to significantly increase delta activity, no medication is currently indicated for this specific purpose.

Medications such as olanzapine and ritanserin are antipsychotics that inhibit serotonin-2 (5-HT) activity and increase SWS. Tiagabine, used as a treatment for partial seizures and panic disorders, increases SWS by acting as a selective GABA reuptake inhibitor. Sodium oxybate, a sodium salt of gamma hydroxybutyric acid utilized for narcolepsy, exerts direct effects on GHB and GABA (B) receptors and enhances SWS. Alprazolam, like most benzodiazepines, is associated with decreased, not enhanced, SWS.

83. Answer: D

EDUCATIONAL OBJECTIVE: Recognize potential causes of recurrent symptoms in patients with obstructive apnea on continuous positive airway pressure (CPAP) therapy.

EXPLANATION: Patients with obstructive sleep apnea (OSA) may develop recurrent symptoms while on CPAP therapy. The initial improvement with CPAP therapy suggests an accurate original diagnosis of apnea. Patient compliance with CPAP may be reduced by the development of rhinosinusitis or mask irritation issues. Technical issues, such as CPAP device malfunction and the development of mask or mouth leaks, may result in subtherapeutic pressures. OSA may also worsen over time following modest weight gain or as an adverse effect of various medications. Occasionally, new conditions may emerge, such as periodic limb movement disorder, depression, or poor sleep hygiene, and also give rise to worsening symptoms.

Patients who do not experience an initial improvement in daytime symptoms must be evaluated more thoroughly. Possible explanations include an incorrect diagnosis of OSA, inadequate therapy, secondary sleep disorders, and depression. In addition, some patients may manifest persistent daytime sleepiness that requires therapy with wake-promoting agents (e.g., modafinil).

84. Answer: A

EDUCATIONAL OBJECTIVE: Understand the role of upper airway muscle activity in sleep-disordered breathing.

EXPLANATION: Upper airway patency is maintained by opposing forces of transmural pressure and airways elastance. Airway tonic activity lessens at sleep onset and predisposes the airway to collapse. Tonic activity, which stabilizes the airway in response to negative intraluminal pressure, is reduced during light sleep but appears more stable in deep sleep.

Patients with obstructive sleep apnea typically have anatomic narrowing of the upper airway that requires increased tonic and phasic activity while awake to maintain patency. With sleep onset, loss of this compensatory tonic activity results in airway collapse. Arousals from apneas–hypopneas cause sleep disruption and further increase the frequency and severity of apneas with the blunted phasic activity seen during the transition from wakefulness to sleep.

85. Answer: B

EDUCATIONAL OBJECTIVE: Recognize the effects of medications on respiratory drive.

EXPLANATION: Opioid use is associated with respiratory depression. Thirty percent of patients on chronic methadone regimens demonstrate central apneas during sleep. Specific mechanisms responsible for opioid-induced central apneas are not well understood. Studies performed during wakefulness demonstrate reduced hypoxic and hypercapnic drives. Theoretically, opioids may also blunt arousal reflexes associated with respiratory events and lengthen the duration of apneas. Therapy is problematic; options include possible narcotic dose reduction, nocturnal oxygen therapy, and the use of bi-level positive airway pressure (BPAP) with a backup rate. Continuous positive airway pressure (CPAP) is typically ineffective. In addition, daytime symptoms may be due to direct sedating properties of the medications, rather than changes in sleep architecture.

Acetazolamide is not associated with central apneas, but rather can be used as a respiratory stimulant. Benzodiazepams (e.g., alprazolam) are unlikely to cause central apneas but may exacerbate obstructive sleep apnea. Digoxin does not affect respiratory drive. The finding of central apneas, particularly with periodic breathing, in a patient on digoxin should prompt an evaluation for decompensated heart failure with increased respiratory drive resulting in central apneas.

86. Answer: B

EDUCATIONAL OBJECTIVE: Recognize known factors associated with sudden infant death syndrome (SIDS).

EXPLANATION: SIDS is the leading cause of death in infants between the age of 1 and 12 months in most industrialized societies. It is defined as the sudden death of an infant under 1 year of age that remains unexplained despite a complete review of clinical history, death scene, and postmortem examination. Specific mechanisms are not well understood. Epidemiologic risk factors for SIDS are known to include endogenous and environmental factors. Endogenous factors include age between 2 and 6 months, prematurity, male gender, and unstable cardiopulmonary control mechanisms. Environmental factors include prenatal maternal smoking or drug abuse, prone sleep position, high room temperature, and sleeping with the face covered. Environmental factors that appear to be protective include breastfeeding, use of pacifiers, and firm bedding.

87. Answer: A

EDUCATIONAL OBJECTIVE: Understand the diagnosis of restless legs syndrome (RLS) in children and adults.

EXPLANATION: For a child between the age of 2 and 12 to be given a diagnosis of RLS, the same four criteria of patterned leg complaints as in the diagnosis of RLS in adults must be present, including a reported description of leg discomfort. If no description can be obtained, then two of three additional findings define RLS, namely, sleep disturbance for age, having a biologic parent or sibling with definite RLS, or polysomnographic evidence of a periodic limb movement (PLM) index of 5 or more per hour. A PLM index of 15 or more is considered significant in adults. A diagnosis of PLM disorder requires a polysomnogram with repetitive movements with precisely defined electromyographic (EMG) findings and clinical sleep disturbance or daytime fatigue.

88. Answer: B

EDUCATIONAL OBJECTIVE: Understand the various behavioral causes of insomnia during childhood.

EXPLANATION: Sleep-onset association disorder typically presents in a child who has problems going to sleep or returning to sleep after an awakening without the presence of specific situations or objects. These associations may include having a parent in the room, being rocked or held, or having a light in the room. Falling asleep is usually an extended process. Treatment is aimed at creating a new set of sleep associations that will allow the child to become a "self-soother" and sleep independently. Children with limit-setting sleep disorder are usually older and have difficulty initiating sleep because of behavioral issues, such as stalling or refusing to go to bed.

89. Answer: C

EDUCATIONAL OBJECTIVE: Recognize the different headache syndromes associated with sleep.

EXPLANATION: Migraine headaches are typified by unilateral throbbing pain with associated symptoms of nausea and photophobia. Migraines are more prevalent in females. Most migraines arise from wakefulness and some may be triggered by sleep deprivation and alleviated by sleep. For patients with nocturnal migraine, the latter arise during REM sleep. Patients with migraine have increased rates of parasomnias.

Cluster headaches are more common in men and demonstrate associated symptoms of orbital pain, lacrimation, rhinorrhea, and possible incomplete Horner syndrome. An association with REM sleep has been suggested for episodic cluster headache.

Hypnic headache is a rare disorder seen in men over age 60 years. It occurs nocturnally and displays no associated autonomic symptoms.

Exploding head syndrome is not associated with pain and is a parasomnia associated with the frightening sensation of a loud noise or explosion occurring within the head, which is experienced during sleep–wake transitions.

90. Answer: C

EDUCATIONAL OBJECTIVE: Understand the significance of sleep–disordered breathing in spinal cord injury (SCI).

EXPLANATION: Patients with SCI have an increased incidence of a variety of sleep complaints, including insomnia, reduced sleep quality, and increased sleep needs. The prevalence of obstructive sleep apnea (OSA) in this population may exceed 40%. Factors that contribute to the development of OSA include increased likelihood of supine sleep position, reduced respiratory capacity, and the use of various antispasmodic and muscle relaxant medications. The severity of OSA does not appear to correlate with the level of spinal cord injury. Apnea may contribute to the disproportionate incidence of nonischemic cardiac deaths in the SCI population. Treatment options may include continuous positive airway pressure (CPAP) if effective with consideration for bi-level positive airway pressure (BiPAP) for refractory respiratory events and hypoventilation.

91. Answer: A

EDUCATIONAL OBJECTIVE: Describe the changes in cardiovascular parameters that occur during sleep.

EXPLANATION: Sympathetic tone decreases and parasympathetic activity increases during NREM sleep compared to wakefulness. These changes in autonomic nervous tone give rise to decreases in heart rate, blood pressure, and cardiac output. Nighttime systolic blood pressure is often about 10% less than that during daytime ("dipping" phenomenon). There are minimal or no changes in stroke volume, peripheral vascular resistance, renal, splanchnic, and skeletal muscle circulation during NREM sleep compared to levels during waking.

Compared to NREM sleep, there is further increase in parasympathetic tone that can result in relative bradycardia and even periods of asystole during tonic REM sleep. In contrast, the higher sympathetic tone during phasic REM sleep causes a higher average heart rate and blood pressure compared to both NREM and tonic REM sleep. Transient increases in heart rate and blood pressure develop during arousals and awakenings due to an enhanced sympathetic tone.

92. Answer: B

EDUCATIONAL OBJECTIVE: Identify the neural systems that contain specific neurotransmitters generating and maintaining the states of wakefulness, NREM sleep, and REM sleep.

EXPLANATION: The main REM sleep neurotransmitter is acetylcholine. Other REM sleep neurotransmitters include gamma aminobutyric acid (GABA) and glycine. On the other hand, hypocretin, histamine, and norepinephrine are involved with the generation of the waking state. Acetylcholine, with neurons in the basal forebrain and laterodorsal tegmentum/pedunculopontine tegmentum, is released during waking and REM sleep, when it causes cortical electroencephalographic (EEG) desynchronization. Wakefulness is associated with the release of certain neurotransmitters located in specific areas of the central nervous system, including histamine (tuberomammillary nucleus of the posterior hypothalamus), hypocretin (perifornical region of the hypothalamus), and norepinephrine (locus coeruleus).

93. Answer: B

EDUCATIONAL OBJECTIVE: Understand the changes in endocrine physiology that occur during sleep.

EXPLANATION: Secretion of hormones oscillates throughout the 24-hour day related either to an endogenous circadian rhythm process or to sleep itself. Of the hormones listed, secretion of cortisol is regulated chiefly by the circadian rhythm. In contrast, growth hormone and prolactin secretion is related to sleep, particularly N3 sleep, and secretion of thyroid-stimulating hormone is influenced by both sleep and circadian processes.

Secretion of cortisol appears to be linked to the circadian rhythm rather than to sleep. Levels of cortisol increase in the early morning, peak at mid-morning, and decline thereafter. The nadir of cortisol levels occurs after the onset of sleep.

Release of growth hormone is linked to sleep, occurring mostly during N3 sleep among adults. However, secretion of growth hormone can also occur in the absence of N3 sleep. There is typically one peak in secretion of growth hormone at sleep onset in men; in contrast, there may be several peaks in growth hormone secretion throughout the day and night in women.

Prolactin secretion increases during N3 sleep and decreases during REM sleep. The circadian rhythm also influences prolactin secretion, with lower hormone levels at noon and higher levels in the evening during wakefulness.

Thyroid-stimulating hormone secretion is linked to both circadian rhythms and sleep. Levels are low during the daytime and progressively increase during the night, with a peak prior to sleep onset. Sleep, itself, inhibits the secretion of thyroid-stimulating hormone.

94. Answer: A

EDUCATIONAL OBJECTIVE: Enumerate the various cytokines and inflammatory mediators that enhance sleep.

EXPLANATION: Several proinflammatory cytokines have been demonstrated to enhance sleep, particularly N3 sleep. These include tumor necrosis factor (TNF-α) and interleukin (IL)-1β; their levels are highest during sleep. In contrast, anti-inflammatory cytokines, such as IL-4, IL-10, and IL-13, inhibit sleep.

Immune processes are also affected by sleep deprivation, with the latter giving rise to increases in IL-1, interferon, and TNF-α. There are also changes in the numbers of T lymphocytes and natural killer cells, lymphocyte mitogenesis and phagocytosis, and circulating immunoglobulins and immune complexes with sleep deprivation.

95. Answer: A

EDUCATIONAL OBJECTIVE: Identify the neural systems that are associated with specific neurotransmitters that control sleep and waking.

EXPLANATION: Dopaminergic neurons are located in the ventral mesencephalic tegmentum and substantia nigra. Dopamine is released during both waking and REM sleep; amphetamines increase its secretion. Other neuronal groups that are associated with sleep–wake neurotransmitters include the tuberomammillary nucleus of the posterior hypothalamus (histamine), locus coeruleus (norepinephrine), and ventrolateral preoptic area (gamma aminobutyric acid [GABA]).

Histamine is released by neurons located in the tuberomammillary nucleus of the posterior hypothalamus during wakefulness. Administration of histamine H-1 receptor blockers increases sleepiness.

Neurons that release norepinephrine are located in the locus coeruleus. Neurotransmitter release occurs during waking, decreases during NREM sleep, and is absent during REM sleep. The ventrolateral preoptic area contains neurons that release GABA, the main central nervous system (CNS) inhibitory neurotransmitter. GABAergic neurons are also located in the thalamus, hypothalamus, basal forebrain, and cerebral cortex. GABA is released during sleep. Benzodiazepines and non-benzodiazepine benzodiazepine receptor agonists (e.g., eszopiclone and zolpidem) act on the GABA-A receptor, whereas sodium oxybate acts on the GABA-B receptor.

96. Answer: C

EDUCATIONAL OBJECTIVE: Describe the changes in thermoregulation that occur during sleep.

EXPLANATION: Sleep affects body temperature and thermoregulation, and a tight coupling exists between sleep–wake circadian rhythms and body temperature. Core body temperature peaks in the late afternoon and early evening, and falls at sleep onset. Minimum core body temperature occurs about 2 hours prior to usual wake time. Activity of cold-sensing neurons decreases during sleep compared to waking. On the other hand, warmth-sensing neurons are more active during sleep onset. Thermoregulation, or the ability to respond to thermal challenges, declines during NREM sleep, and diminishes further during REM sleep. Although sweating and shivering are still present during NREM sleep, shivering is absent during REM sleep. Sleep onset typically occurs during the declining phase of the temperature rhythm, and initiating sleep during the falling phase of the temperature rhythm generally results in a shorter sleep-onset latency, greater total sleep time, and increase in stage N3 sleep. Conversely, initiating sleep during the rising phase of the temperature rhythm is associated with a more prolonged sleep-onset latency, reduced total sleep time, and diminished stage N3 sleep. Awakening typically occurs during the rising phase of the temperature rhythm following the temperature nadir.

97. Answer: A

EDUCATIONAL OBJECTIVE: Distinguish the different sleep stages based on new sleep scoring criteria recommended by the *2007 American Academy of Sleep Medicine Manual for the Scoring of Sleep and Associated Events.*

EXPLANATION: The American Academy of Sleep Medicine has proposed new criteria for sleep stage scoring in 2007. Similar to the Rechtschaffen and Kales sleep scoring system, sleep stages are scored in 30-second epochs; each epoch is assigned a sleep stage that comprises the greatest percentage of the epoch.

On the basis of their recommendations, NREM stage 1 (N1) sleep among adults is defined by the presence of low-amplitude, mixed-frequency (4 to 7 Hz) waves that have replaced alpha electroencephalographic waves and occupy greater than 50% of the epoch. In individuals who do not generate alpha waves, stage N1 sleep is characterized by the start of 4 to 7 Hz waves with slowing of background activity by at least 1 Hz compared to wakefulness; vertex sharp waves with duration of less than 0.5 seconds that are maximal over the central regions; or slow eye movements.

For children (≥2 months postterm), stage N1 is present when the dominant posterior electroencephalographic rhythm is replaced by low-amplitude, mixed-frequency (4 to 7 Hz) waves, occupying >50% of the epoch. In children who do not generate a dominant posterior rhythm, the start of stage N1 sleep is determined by the presence of 4 to 7 Hz waves with slowing of the background activity by at least 1 to 2 Hz compared to wakefulness; vertex sharp waves; slow eye movements; rhythmic anterior theta activity; hypnagogic hypersynchrony; or diffuse or occipital predominant high-amplitude 3- to 5-Hz rhythmic activity.

Reference:

Iber C, Ancoli-Israel S, Chesson A, et al. for the American Academy of Sleep Medicine. *The AASM Manual for the Scoring of Sleep and Associated Events: Rules, Terminology and Technical Specifications.* 1st ed. Westchester, Ill: American Academy of Sleep Medicine; 2007.

98. Answer: D

EDUCATIONAL OBJECTIVE: Identify the recommended and alternative sensors for respiratory events based on the *2007 American Academy of Sleep Medicine Manual for the Scoring of Sleep and Associated Events.*

EXPLANATION: In 2007, the American Academy of Sleep Medicine provided recommendations for the scoring of sleep stages, arousals, and sleep-related events (i.e., respiratory, cardiac, and movement). The recommended sensor for detecting apneas is the oronasal thermal sensor. Alternative sensors for apneas include nasal air pressure transducer, end tidal Pco_2, or summed calibrated inductance plethysmography (for children). For hypopneas, nasal air pressure transducer is the recommended sensor, and inductance plethysmography or oronasal thermal sensor are acceptable alternatives. Esophageal manometry or inductance plethysmography are the recommended sensors for respiratory effort.

Among adults, an apnea is defined by a decrease in peak thermal sensor amplitude by at least 90% from baseline for a duration of at least 10 seconds (≥90% of the duration of each event must meet the criteria for minimum thermal sensor amplitude reduction from baseline). It can be further classified as an obstructive event if inspiratory effort is present throughout the entire period; a central event if inspiratory effort is absent throughout the entire period; or a mixed event if absent inspiratory effort in the initial part of the period is followed by the presence of inspiratory effort.

A hypopnea among adults, on the other hand, is characterized by a reduction in oronasal pressure by at least 30% of baseline for a duration of at least 10 seconds accompanied by at least a 4% oxygen desaturation (≥90% of the duration of each event must meet the criteria for minimum nasal pressure amplitude reduction from baseline).

Finally, a respiratory effort–related arousal is present when breaths are associated with increasing respiratory efforts or flattening of the nasal pressure waveform with a duration of at least 10 seconds and preceding an arousal, but not meeting criteria for either apnea or hypopnea.

Reference:

Iber C, Ancoli-Israel S, Chesson A, et al. for the American Academy of Sleep Medicine. *The AASM Manual for the Scoring of Sleep and Associated Events: Rules, Terminology and Technical Specifications.* 1st ed. Westchester, Ill: American Academy of Sleep Medicine; 2007.

99. Answer: D

EDUCATIONAL OBJECTIVE: Determine which measures are effective in increasing alertness and decreasing sleepiness during night shift work.

EXPLANATION: Shift work may take several forms, including permanent night hours or rotating schedules. Not every shift worker develops sleep disturbance and excessive sleepiness at work (shift work sleep disorder). There appears to be individual differences in the ability to tolerate shift work, and some workers can adapt more readily to nonconventional work and sleep hours than others. Shift work sleep disorder can pose a significant hazard in the work environment, and decreased alertness and vigilance resulting from circadian changes in levels of alertness and sleep deprivation from poor daytime sleep quality can give rise to work-related physical injuries, accidents, and impaired work performance. Persons with shift work sleep disorder may present with complaints of chronic fatigue and malaise as well as a variety of nonspecific gastrointestinal (dyspepsia), cardiovascular (ischemic heart disease), and endocrine (decreased glucose tolerance) disturbances.

Intermittent exposure to bright lights in the workplace (and restriction of light exposure during the morning trip home from work), administration of psychostimulants (e.g., caffeine or modafinil) during evening work hours, and scheduled napping can enhance alertness and reduce sleepiness. Use of hypnotic agents or melatonin following night shift can enhance sleep quality during daytime sleep, but does not significantly or consistently improve alertness and performance during night shift work. Scheduling phase delays in shifts (night to day to evening) is preferable to phase advances in shift schedules.

100. Answer: C

EDUCATIONAL OBJECTIVE: Describe the proper performance of the maintenance of wakefulness test (MWT).

EXPLANATION: The MWT measures a person's ability to remain awake for a defined time in quiet situations. It may also be used to assess response to treatment in patients with excessive sleepiness. The 40-minute protocol is preferred over the 20-minute protocol when assessing an individual's ability to remain awake or when an inability to remain awake represents a public or personal safety issue.

The recommended protocol consists of four nap opportunities, each 40 minutes in duration, that are performed at 2-hour intervals in a dark, quiet room. The first nap trial is started about 1.5 to 3 hours after the patient's customary wake time. The patient is asked to sit in bed in a semireclined position with the back and head supported by a bed rest. Whether or not sleep logs are used or a PSG is to be performed prior to the test should be individualized as determined by the clinician.

Patients are instructed to sit still, look directly while avoiding the light, and try to stay awake during the test. Measures to stay awake such as singing are not allowed. Standard biocalibrations are performed before each trial. A light breakfast is provided 1 hour before the first trial, and lunch is given immediately after the second trial. Bathroom trips, if needed, are scheduled prior to each trial. The use of tobacco, caffeine, and stimulant agents should be avoided. Room temperature should be adjusted on the basis of the patient's level of comfort.

The test is terminated once unequivocal sleep (defined as three consecutive epochs of stage 1 sleep, or one epoch of any other sleep stage) occurs, or after 40 minutes if no sleep is recorded. Drug screening may be considered. Mean sleep latency less than 8 minutes on the 40-minute MWT is considered abnormal. Values greater than 8 minutes but less than 40 minutes are of uncertain significance. Staying awake on all trials may provide an appropriate expectation for individuals who require the highest level of alertness for safety.

Reference:

Standards of Practice Committee of the American Academy of Sleep Medicine (AASM). Practice parameters for clinical use of the multiple sleep latency test and the maintenance of wakefulness test. *Sleep.* 2005; 28(1):113–121.

101. Answer: D

EDUCATIONAL OBJECTIVE: Identify the various cardiac rhythm abnormalities that may be encountered during polysomnography.

EXPLANATION: The *2007 American Academy of Sleep Medicine Manual for the Scoring of Sleep and Associated Events* provided definitions of some of the common cardiac rhythm abnormalities that may be encountered during polysomnography. *Atrial fibrillation* is characterized by an irregularly irregular rhythm with no distinct P waves. Cardiac pause >3 seconds for patients 6 years and older defines an *asystole. Bradycardia* is present if the heart rate (HR) is less than 40 beats per minute (for patients 6 years and older). The cardiac rhythm is considered *sinus tachycardia* if the HR is greater than 90 beats per minute for adult patients; sinus rates are faster in children compared to adults. Finally, *wide-complex tachycardia* or *narrow-complex tachycardia* is defined by an HR greater than 100 beats per minute, with at least three consecutive beats with QRS duration at least 120 ms or less than 120 ms, respectively.

In the Sleep Heart Health Study, individuals with sleep-disordered breathing had four times the odds of atrial fibrillation compared with those without sleep-disordered breathing. In addition, the recurrence rate of atrial fibrillation after successful cardioversion is higher in patients with untreated obstructive sleep apnea.

References:

1. Iber C, Ancoli-Israel S, Chesson A, et al. for the American Academy of Sleep Medicine. *The AASM Manual for the Scoring of Sleep and Associated Events: Rules, Terminology and Technical Specifications.* 1st ed. Westchester, Ill: American Academy of Sleep Medicine; 2007.
2. Kanagala R, Murali NS, Friedman PA, et al. Obstructive sleep apnea and the recurrence of atrial fibrillation. *Circulation.* 2003; 107:2589–2594.
3. Mehra R, Benjamin EJ, Shahar E, et al. Association of nocturnal arrhythmias with sleep-disordered breathing: The Sleep Heart Health Study. *Am J Respir Crit Care Med.* 2006; 173:910–916.

102. Answer: D

EDUCATIONAL OBJECTIVE: Describe the developmental electrophysiologic milestones of the different polysomnographic parameters.

EXPLANATION: Sleep spindles commonly first appear after 4 weeks to 3 months of age, whereas K-complexes appear first after 6 months of age. Slow-wave activity is first evident at 8 to 12 weeks of age. Distinct electroencephalographic (EEG) features that allow differentiation of NREM sleep into three specific stages (i.e., N1, N2, and N3) develop at 3 to 6 months of age.

Sleep among newborns is polyphasic, occurring several times throughout the 24-hour day, and typically becomes monophasic after 3 to 5 years of age. In addition, newborn infants generally sleep about 70% during a 24-hour day, whereas adults spend about 25% to 35% of the 24-hour day sleeping. In the first 6 months of life, sleep is classified into active sleep (REM sleep equivalent), quiet sleep (NREM sleep equivalent), and indeterminate sleep or transitional sleep. After 6 months of age, sleep stages are classified using the conventional adult criteria of NREM sleep (stages N1, N2, or N3) and REM sleep.

103. Answer: C

EDUCATIONAL OBJECTIVE: Describe the changes in sleep architecture associated with the administration of antidepressants.

EXPLANATION: Tricyclic antidepressants, such as amitriptyline, clomipramine, desipramine, protriptyline, and trimipramine, act by inhibiting the uptake of norepinephrine and serotonin, and blocking the activity of histamine and acetylcholine. Whereas tertiary amines, such as amitriptyline, clomipramine, doxepin, and imipramine, are sedating (decreasing sleep-onset latency and increasing both total sleep time and sleep efficiency), the secondary amines including protriptyline are relatively alerting (prolonging sleep-onset latency and decreasing sleep efficiency). Most tricyclic antidepressants increase REM sleep latency and decrease REM sleep. Trimipramine use has not been shown to change REM sleep significantly. Nefazodone, a serotonin antagonist and reuptake inhibitor, is associated with increased REM sleep.

104. Answer: B

EDUCATIONAL OBJECTIVE: Describe the role of bright light therapy for delayed sleep phase disorder (DSPD).

EXPLANATION: DSPD is characterized by a habitually delayed nocturnal sleep period that occurs later than the desired bedtime. Individuals are commonly unable to fall asleep until the early morning hours (between 1:00 a.m. and 6:00 a.m.) and have difficulty waking until late morning or early afternoon (between 11:00 a.m. and 2:00 p.m.). However, they typically have no difficulty remaining asleep following the onset of sleep. Prevalence of DSPD is highest among adolescents and young adults, with a mean age of onset of about 20 years. Diagnosis is usually based mainly on history and sleep diaries. Actigraphy performed for several days reveals a stable delay of the habitual sleep period. Polysomnography is not routinely indicated for the diagnosis of DSPD.

Appropriately timed exposure to bright light is an effective therapy for DSPD. Morning exposure to bright lights, preferably after the core body temperature nadir (CTmin), produces a phase advance in the sleep–wake circadian cycle.

The body temperature nadir is often about 1 to 2 hours after the habitual mid-sleep time. However, light administered prior to the temperature nadir could further phase delay circadian rhythms. Evening avoidance of bright light is also important. Phototherapy should not be used in patients with retinopathy or photosensitivity and should be avoided in those with bipolar disorder, in whom it may precipitate a hypomanic state.

Reference:

Chesson AL, Littner M, Davida D, et al. Practice parameters for the use of light therapy in the treatment of sleep disorders. *Sleep*. 1999; 22(5):641–660.

105. Answer: D

EDUCATIONAL OBJECTIVE: Describe the clinical features of jet lag.

EXPLANATION: Jet lag is characterized by transient sleep disturbance (i.e., insomnia or excessive sleepiness) following rapid eastward or westward air travel across multiple time zones because the traveler's endogenous circadian rhythm remains temporarily aligned to the home time zone and has not synchronized to the new local time zone. Individuals traveling westward are phase-advanced relative to the new clock time, and thus present with early evening sleepiness as well as increased wakefulness during the early morning hours. In contrast, those traveling eastward are phase-delayed and generally complain of difficulty falling asleep and difficulty awakening the next day.

The severity of symptoms tend to be worse with greater amounts of time zone transitions, as well as following eastward travel compared to westbound travel. Symptoms typically remit spontaneously after 2 to 3 days, but may last longer with eastbound travel. If treatment is desired, appropriately timed exposure to bright lights (evening exposure after westward travel and morning exposure after eastward travel) might hasten synchronization to the new time zone.

106. Answer: C

EDUCATIONAL OBJECTIVE: Identify the ages at which developmental sleep behavior milestones occur in children.

EXPLANATION: There is great individual variability in the ages at which developmental sleep milestones develop in a child. Prior to 6 weeks, sleep periods occur randomly throughout the 24-hour day. At 6 weeks, the longest sleep period starts to occur at night. Consolidation of daytime sleep into discrete naps develops at 3 months, and nocturnal sleep consolidation with ability to sleep through the night is present between 6 and 9 months. By 3 to 5 years, daytime napping ceases. Most children develop a circadian sleep phase preference ("eveningness" vs. "morningness") between 6 and 12 years of age. Adolescents (between 12 and 18 years of age) may begin to acquire a phase delay in their sleep schedules.

107. Answer: B

EDUCATIONAL OBJECTIVE: Describe the various factors that may be associated with the generation and maintenance of insomnia.

EXPLANATION: In Speilman's model, factors related to the genesis and persistence of sleep disturbance can be classified into *predisposing factors* that are present before the start of insomnia and that increase the likelihood of developing insomnia (physiologic and psychologic hyperarousal, or genetic predisposition), *precipitating factors* that trigger the start of insomnia (acute stress, abrupt alterations in sleep–wake schedules, illness, or substance or medication use), and *perpetuating factors* that sustain sleep disturbance and contribute to the persistence of insomnia independent of the precipitating causes (maladaptive sleep–wake behaviors, poor sleep hygiene, and unrealistic expectations about sleep).

Reference:

Spielman AJ, Caruso LS, Glovinski PB. A behavioral perspective on insomnia treatment. *Psychiatr Clin North Am.* 1987; 10:541–553.

108. Answer: B

EDUCATIONAL OBJECTIVE: Distinguish among the various behavioral therapies for insomnia.

EXPLANATION: The objectives of behavioral therapy for insomnia include curtailing physical and psychic influences that may disrupt sleep onset and maintenance, and encouraging activities that are conducive to sleep and that regularize sleep–wake schedules.

Sleep restriction, by promoting a state of relative sleep deprivation, is designed to improve sleep efficiency and shorten sleep latency. Patients, especially those who spend considerable time in bed awake, are instructed to limit time in bed only to actual sleep time by progressively delaying or advancing bedtimes with a goal of maintaining a sleep efficiency (the percentage of time in bed spent sleeping [total sleep time/time in bed] $\times$ 100%) between about 80% and 90%, until a desired sleep duration is reached. Wake up time is kept constant and naps are not allowed. A closely related technique is temporal control, which entails a constancy in the sleep–wake schedule by asking the patient to get out of bed at the same time each day and to refrain from napping. Finally, paradoxical intention is designed to decrease the anxiety associated with unsuccessful efforts to fall asleep by instructing patients with insomnia to go to bed and to try to stay awake as long as they possibly can rather than trying to sleep.

109. Answer: D

EDUCATIONAL OBJECTIVE: Describe the clinical features of psychophysiologic insomnia.

EXPLANATION: Psychophysiologic insomnia is a chronic cause of sleep disturbance. The onset of insomnia may be related to an identifiable stressor, but the sleep disturbance persists even after resolution of the latter due to the development of maladaptive learned sleep-preventing behaviors as well as heightened conditioned cognitive and physiologic arousal responses. Although patients may express anxiety about their inability to sleep better, excessive worry and concern do not pervade other aspects of daily livening, as is the case with generalized anxiety disorder. Because they have developed a conditioned arousal to their own bed and bedroom, patients may, surprisingly, sleep better when they try to sleep in any room other than their bedroom, such as in the sleep laboratory (reverse first-night effect). Sleep also commences more readily when patients are not trying "too hard" to fall asleep, or when they are distracted during their habitual bedtime. Psychophysiologic insomnia accounts for about 15% of cases of chronic insomnia and affects women more often than men. Diagnosis is based on a compatible clinical history and seldom requires polysomnography. If polysomnography is performed for other indications, subjective report of sleep time is often less, and duration of sleep-onset latency is commonly longer than objective measures.

110. Answer: D

EDUCATIONAL OBJECTIVE: Identify the causative agent of sleeping sickness.

EXPLANATION: Sleeping sickness is caused by the protozoan *Trypanosoma brucei* or *Trypanosoma rhodesiense,* which is endemic in certain regions of intertropical Africa. It is transmitted via the bite of a tsetse fly. There are two stages of human disease, namely, an early hemolymphatic stage with fever, adenopathy, skin lesions, facial edema, and cardiac arrhythmias, and a later meningoencephalitic stage when neurologic symptoms, including excessive sleepiness, headaches, sensory deficits, and abnormal reflexes, emerge. Although patients generally present with excessive sleepiness and insomnia, reversal of the sleep–wake periods is not uncommon. Polysomnography may demonstrate a scarcity of vertex sharp waves, spindles and K-complexes, and sleep-onset REM periods. Diagnosis requires demonstration of the infecting organisms in blood, bone marrow, lymph node aspirates, or cerebrospinal fluid. Sleep disturbance can be reversed by successful antiparasitic therapy.

Reference:

Sanner BM, Buchner N, Kotterba S, et al. Polysomnography in acute African trypanosomiasis. *J Neurol.* 2000; 247:878–879.

111. Answer: B

EDUCATIONAL OBJECTIVE: Describe the clinical features of narcolepsy without cataplexy.

EXPLANATION: Narcolepsy is a neurologic disorder characterized by excessive daytime sleepiness. Abnormal manifestations of REM sleep physiology, such as cataplexy (abrupt, transient, and bilateral loss or reduction of postural muscle tone occurring during wakefulness that is precipitated by intense emotion such as laughter), sleep paralysis (transient loss of the ability to move occurring at sleep onset [hypnagogic] or upon awakening [hypnopompic]), and sleep hallucinations, may be present. However, only about 10% to 15% of patients demonstrate the full clinical tetrad of excessive sleepiness, cataplexy, sleep paralysis, and sleep hallucinations. Other common features of narcolepsy include automatic behavior, nocturnal sleep disturbance, and altered dreams.

There are several clinical subtypes of narcolepsy including 1) narcolepsy without cataplexy, 2) narcolepsy with cataplexy with normal hypocretin-1 levels in the cerebrospinal fluid (CSF) (up to 10% of cases), and 3) isolated cataplexy.

Narcolepsy without cataplexy, as its name implies, is not associated with cataplexy. It accounts for about 10% to 50% of cases of narcolepsy.

Sleep paralysis, sleep hallucinations, and cataplexy-like symptoms, such as prolonged episodes of tiredness related to atypical triggers (exercise, stress, or sex), may be present. CSF levels of hypocretin-1 are generally normal in HLA DQB1*0602-negative narcolepsy without cataplexy patients, but low hypocretin-1 levels (<110 pg/ml) are present in up to 10% to 20% of cases of HLA DQB1*0602-positive narcolepsy without cataplexy and in 20% of cases of narcolepsy with cataplexy-like or atypical episodes.

112. Answer: A

EDUCATIONAL OBJECTIVE: Enumerate the differences in the clinical features between narcolepsy and idiopathic hypersomnia.

EXPLANATION: In patients with idiopathic hypersomnia, sleepiness is generally severe and constant, occurring even after sufficient or increased amounts of nighttime sleep. Sleepiness occurs without any identifiable cause. Compared to narcolepsy, daytime naps are typically longer but unrefreshing in idiopathic hypersomnia. Although cataplexy is distinctively absent, patients with idiopathic hypersomnia may have episodes of sleep paralysis and hypnagogic hallucinations. There is less predictable improvement in sleepiness with stimulant therapy compared to narcolepsy.

Polysomnographic features include a normal sleep architecture, and sleep duration may be either normal (*idiopathic hypersomnia without long sleep time* with a sleep duration of greater than 6 hours but less than 10 hours) or prolonged (*idiopathic hypersomnia with long sleep time* with a sleep duration of at least 10 hours, often 12 to 14 hours). Multiple sleep latency testing generally reveals a short sleep-onset latency without sleep-onset REM periods. HLA CW2 positivity may be present in idiopathic hypersomnia, rather than DQB1*0602 positivity, which is more common in narcolepsy. Cerebrospinal fluid levels of hypocretin-1 are normal.

113. Answer: A

EDUCATIONAL OBJECTIVE: Describe the association between narcolepsy and specific human leukocyte antigens (HLAs), namely DR2 and DQ1.

EXPLANATION: Certain HLAs are more prevalent in patients with narcolepsy, including DR2 (particularly the subtype DR15) and DQ1 (in particular DQ6 [DQB1*0602]). The prevalence of DR2 in subjects with narcolepsy varies among different populations (100% among Japanese, 90% to 95% in Caucasians, and 60% in African Americans). HLA DQB1*0602 is present in 90% of patients with narcolepsy with cataplexy, but is less common in those without cataplexy (40% to 60%). DQB1*0602 positivity also appears to be associated with both frequency and severity of cataplexy. Most multiplex family cases (multiple members of the family with narcolepsy) are HLA DQB1*0602 positive. However, HLA typing has limited diagnostic utility since most persons positive for HLA DQB1*0602 do not have narcolepsy. Furthermore, a negative test result does not exclude the diagnosis of narcolepsy because about 1% to 5% of all patients with narcolepsy are negative for DQB1*0602.

114. Answer: A

EDUCATIONAL OBJECTIVE: Describe the differences between nightmares and sleep terrors.

EXPLANATION: Nightmares are unpleasant and frightening dreams that occur during REM sleep. Episodes typically occur during the latter half of the night. Following awakening from a nightmare, the individual is awake and alert. There is full recall of the preceding dream. Return to sleep is delayed.

Nightmares have to be distinguished from sleep terrors, which are more likely to occur during the first half of the night following awakenings from stage N3 sleep. During episodes of sleep terrors, individuals are commonly confused and disoriented, have partial or complete amnesia of the events, and have no difficulty with returning back to sleep. Associated clinical features of sleep terrors include inconsolability, misperception of the environment, ambulation, vocalizations, and intense autonomic activation, such as tachypnea, tachycardia, elevated blood pressure, papillary dilatation, and diaphoresis.

115. Answer: C

EDUCATIONAL OBJECTIVE: Describe the clinical features of sleep enuresis.

EXPLANATION: Sleep enuresis is defined as recurrent involuntary bed-wetting occurring during sleep after 5 years of age. Children develop the ability to postpone voiding in response to a full bladder, initially during wakefulness and eventually during sleep as well, by 18 months to 3 years of age. Sleep enuresis can be classified as either primary (episodes occur at least twice a week in children older than 5 years of age who have never been consistently dry during sleep) or secondary (episodes recur at least twice a week for at least 3 months after the child or adult has maintained dryness for at least 6 consecutive months).

An organic etiology should be considered if urgency, an abnormality in urinary flow, or involuntary voiding during wakefulness is present. The spontaneous cure rate in children with primary sleep enuresis is about 5% annually.

Treatment consists of pharmacotherapy (desmopressin or tricyclic antidepressants for specific situations that require acute control, such as during sleepovers) or behavioral therapy (enuresis alarm system or bladder training exercises). Secondary causes of enuresis should be properly corrected.

116. Answer: D

EDUCATIONAL OBJECTIVE: Identify the factors that increase the risk of high-altitude periodic breathing.

EXPLANATION: Cycles of central apneas and hyperpneas can develop acutely on ascent to high altitude, usually greater than 4,000 m. Relative hypoxia at altitude will result in reflex hyperventilation, which, in turn, will give rise to hypocapnic alkalosis and central apnea. The rising $PaCO_2$ during the apneic episode will eventually trigger the resumption of ventilation, and the cycle repeats itself. Periodic breathing occurs during NREM sleep; respiration stabilizes during REM sleep. Symptoms, including frequent awakenings, nocturnal dyspnea, sleepiness and fatigue, tend to be more severe with extreme elevation, speedier ascent, male gender, and in persons with increased hypoxic ventilatory chemoresponsiveness. Periodic breathing generally improves over time with adaptation unless elevation is extreme. Therapy, if necessary, involves descent from altitude, oxygen therapy, or administration of acetazolamide.

117. Answer: C

EDUCATIONAL OBJECTIVE: Describe the pathogenetic mechanisms related to nocturnal asthma.

EXPLANATION: Nocturnal bronchoconstriction among patients with asthma may give rise to frequent awakenings due to coughing, dyspnea and chest discomfort, insomnia, and excessive sleepiness. Sleep fragmentation can develop with a decrease in sleep efficiency and total sleep time as well as a greater wake time after sleep onset. Sleep-related hypoxemia can occur, especially during acute attacks of bronchospasm or in advanced disease. Many factors contribute to the pathogenesis of nocturnal bronchoconstriction in patients with asthma, including an endogenous circadian variability in airflow (lowest levels occur in the early morning), sleep-related changes in lung volumes and flow rates, and alterations in autonomic nervous system activity (i.e., increased parasympathetic tone and decreased sympathetic tone), hormone levels (cortisol), and inflammatory mediators (bronchoalveolar lavage total leukocyte count, neutrophils, and eosinophils). Nocturnal gastroesophageal reflux (GER) can worsen nighttime asthma control. Finally, both snoring and obstructive sleep apnea can worsen upper airway obstruction and increase the frequency of nocturnal asthma attacks in persons with both conditions.

Reference:

Ciftci TU, Ciftci B, Guven SF, et al. Effect of nasal continuous positive airway pressure in uncontrolled nocturnal asthmatic patients with obstructive sleep apnea syndrome. *Respir Med.* 2005; 99:529–534.

118. Answer: C

EDUCATIONAL OBJECTIVE: Describe the changes in sleep associated with human immunodeficiency virus (HIV) infection.

EXPLANATION: Complaints of insomnia, frequent awakenings, and excessive sleepiness are not uncommon in patients with HIV disease.

Sleep disturbance may be due directly to the infection and HIV-related symptoms (impaired functional status [lower T cell counts] is associated with worse sleep quality), an underlying encephalopathy, the development of depression and anxiety, or antiviral therapy for HIV infection (both efavirenz and zidovudine can give rise to insomnia). Polysomnography may demonstrate a decrease in sleep latency, decrease in sleep efficiency, and increase in frequency of arousals in these patients. A decrease in stage N2 and N3 sleep may develop during advanced disease.

119. Answer: B

EDUCATIONAL OBJECTIVE: Enumerate the differences between childhood and adult obstructive sleep apnea.

EXPLANATION: Obstructive sleep apnea in children differs from the disorder involving adults in several ways. Excessive sleepiness is more common among adult patients compared to children, in whom behavioral problems, such as hyperactivity and restlessness, are more likely to be encountered. Whereas adult cases of obstructive sleep apnea are more often seen among men, there is no significant gender difference in prevalence among children. Polysomnography may demonstrate a normal sleep architecture, with few respiratory event-related arousals and less severe oxygen desaturation in children. Adults, on the other hand, may have reductions in stages N3 and REM sleep, more frequent arousals, and greater oxygen desaturation.

Adenotonsillar enlargement is an important risk factor for childhood obstructive sleep apnea, and adenotonsillectomy, rather than continuous positive airway pressure therapy, is the first-line and most common therapy for children with this disorder. Polysomnography is recommended following adenotonsillectomy to assess the efficacy of the procedure in children with complicated cases of obstructive sleep apnea (i.e., craniofacial abnormalities). Continuous positive airway pressure therapy may be considered for children when adenotonsillectomy is not indicated or contraindicated; when significant symptoms persist following adenotonsillectomy; and during the perioperative period in children with severe disease. When continuous positive airway pressure therapy is chosen, periodic titration may be considered to account for the age-related changes in upper airway and craniofacial dimensions. Finally, oral devices may be used in older adolescents when growth of their craniofacial bones and upper airway soft tissues is largely complete.

120. Answer: A

EDUCATIONAL OBJECTIVE: Describe the clinical features of limit-setting sleep disorder.

EXPLANATION: Limit-setting sleep disorder is characterized by repetitive refusal by a child to go to sleep at an age-appropriate time when requested to do so because of inadequate enforcement of bedtimes by the caregiver. The child often stalls going to bed by asking to be read to in bed, to be allowed to watch a few minutes more of television or to play, or to have something to drink or eat. Sleep comes naturally and quickly if the caretaker recognizes the child's attempts to delay his or her bedtime and when limits to further activity are strictly enforced.

The clinical history is not consistent with either psychophysiologic insomnia, in which learned sleep-preventing associations and conditioned arousal to the bedroom environment give rise to insomnia, or delayed sleep phase syndrome, which is a circadian sleep–wake rhythm disorder characterized by a habitual delay in the major nocturnal sleep period with late bedtimes and equally late waking times. Lastly, children with sleep-onset association disorder are unable to fall asleep on their own in the absence of certain desired, but inappropriate, conditions or objects (e.g., feeding bottle, favorite doll, or being held by a caregiver).

121. Answer: A

EDUCATIONAL OBJECTIVE: Understand the relationship between sleep fragmentation and sleep deprivation.

EXPLANATION: In experimental studies of sleep fragmentation, frequent brief arousals, even in the absence of visual electroencephalographic (EEG) changes, subjects were sleepier the following day. Sleepiness is more closely related to sleep fragmentation than to sleep stage parameters. Hormones, respiration, and performance measures are similarly affected by sleep derivation and sleep fragmentation. In addition, the impact of sleep fragmentation diminishes as the interval between arousals increases (i.e., sleep can have restorative effects when the interval between arousals is greater than 10 minutes).

Reference:

Bonnet MH. Infrequent periodic sleep disruption: effects on sleep, performance and mood. *Physiol Behav.* 1989; 45:1049–1055.

122. Answer: B

EDUCATIONAL OBJECTIVE: Learn indications for actigraphy.

EXPLANATION: Actigraphy is a small motion-sensing device usually worn on the wrist. The small size of the device and inexpensive nature of the test allow prolonged monitoring for several days or weeks. Actigraphy is superior to sleep logs in detecting brief arousals during the night. Since actigraphy identifies sleep and wake on motion, it can underestimate sleep if an individual is in bed awake but motionless, a situation more commonly seen in elderly patients and depressed individuals. Actigraphy is an ideal tool to measure circadian rhythm sleep disturbances, such as shift work, because it can be worn for an extended period of time and in a field setting.

Reference:

Ancoli-Israel S. Actigraphy. In: Kryger MH, Roth T, Dement WC, eds. *Principles and Practice of Sleep Medicine.* 4th ed. Philadelphia, Pa: Elsevier; 2005:1459–1467.

123. Answer: C

EDUCATIONAL OBJECTIVE: Understand gastric physiology during sleep.

EXPLANATION: Reflux events may occur during sleep but the majority of events occur during brief awakenings from sleep. When they occur during sleep, they are most likely to do so during stage 2 sleep.

Reference:

Freidin N, Fisher MJ, Taylor W, et al. Sleep and nocturnal acid reflux in normal subjects and patients with reflux esophagitis. *Gut.* 1991; 32:1275–1279.

124. Answer: B

EDUCATIONAL OBJECTIVE: Characterize dreaming in persons with posttraumatic stress disorder (PTSD).

EXPLANATION: Dreams reported by healthy persons frequently contain elements of recent experiences but the events rarely correspond to actual events. In contrast, there is a tendency for dreams occurring in persons suffering from PTSD to contain unaltered memories of traumatic events. Polysomnographic studies of these dreams have not been consistent but it now appears that the majority of PTSD dreams arise out of REM sleep, though they can occur from N1 and N2 as well. There is no evidence for a lack of atonia in these dreams or that they are more easily recalled.

Reference:

Mellman TA, Pigeon WR. Dreams and nightmares in post-traumatic stress disorder. In: Kryger MH, Roth T, Dement WC, eds. *Principles and Practice of Sleep Medicine.* 4th ed. Philadelphia, Pa: Elsevier; 2005:573–578.

125. Answer: C

EDUCATIONAL OBJECTIVE: Identify the effects of medications on sleep architecture.

EXPLANATION: Most antidepressant medications are REM suppressants. The hypnogram in this question shows a normal amount of stage N3 sleep but a delayed and decreased stage REM sleep. Benzodiazepines are potent stage N3 suppressors but milder REM sleep suppressors. The non-benzodiazepine hypnotic agents are not strong stage REM or N3 sleep suppressors. One study found that women taking oral contraceptives showed shorter REM latency, more total REM sleep time, and less stage N3 sleep than women who are not taking the medication.

Reference:

Burdick RS, Hoffmann R, Armitage R. Short note: oral contraceptives and sleep in depressed and healthy women. *Sleep.* 2002; 25(3):347–349.

126. Answer: D

EDUCATIONAL OBJECTIVE: Describe the relationship between insomnia and mood disorders.

EXPLANATION: Longitudinal studies on the relationship between insomnia and mental illness have found that, while insomnia associated with psychiatric disorders has classically been defined as "secondary insomnia," there is now a general agreement that the term "comorbid insomnia" more accurately describes the relationship between the two. Breslau et al. looked at the relationship between insomnia and the onset of a new psychiatric illness in a longitudinal study over 3.5 years. A greater incidence of new psychiatric illness was associated with a history of insomnia; new-onset major depression occurred in 15.9% of the population with a history of insomnia versus only 4.6% of those without a history of insomnia. In addition, insomnia often precedes the onset of symptoms of a mood disorder, particularly during relapse. In one study, insomnia appeared before the onset of mood disorder in 41% of cases and before a relapse in 56% of cases. Successful treatment of a mood disorder does not guarantee improvement in the sleep complaint. Insomnia is often the most common residual symptom (44%) following remission of depression. Finally, many new antidepressants, such as the selective serotonin reuptake inhibitors, tend to be activating and can often cause sleep disturbance while at the same time they are improving mood.

References:

1. NIH State-of-the-Science Conference Statement. Manifestations and management of chronic insomnia in adults. Bethesda, Md; August 18, 2005:1–18.
2. Breslau N, Roth T, Rosenthal L, et al. Sleep disturbance and psychiatric disorders: a longitudinal epidemiological study of young adults. *Biol Psychiatry.* 1996; 39:411–418.
3. Ohayon MM, Roth T. Place of chronic insomnia in the course of depressive and anxiety disorders. *J Psychiatr Res.* 2003; 37:9–15.
4. Nierenberg AA, Keefe BR, Leslie VC, et al. Residual symptoms in depressed patients who respond acutely to fluoxetine. *J Clin Psychiatry.* 1999; 60:221–225.

127. Answer: A

EDUCATIONAL OBJECTIVE: Understanding behavioral interventions for insomnia.

EXPLANATION: Patients with insomnia often underestimate their total sleep time. Limiting their time in bed to their average subjective sleep time results in a state of mild sleep deprivation. Sleep deprivation, in turn, increases the homeostatic drive to sleep, resulting in a shorter sleep-onset latency and decreased number and duration of awakenings during sleep. Delaying bedtime can cause a realignment of the bedtime with the underlying circadian rhythm, but this is not the primary goal of sleep restriction therapy.

128. Answer: B

EDUCATIONAL OBJECTIVE: Characterize the effect of alcohol on sleep.

EXPLANATION: Acute use of alcohol in nonalcoholics can hasten sleep onset and increase NREM sleep including stage N3 sleep. It will also suppress REM sleep in a dose-dependent manner during the first half of the night. An adult can metabolize about 10 ml of 100% alcohol per hour regardless of blood alcohol concentration. Metabolism may be complete within 4 to 5 hours after consumption. Thus, the latter portion of the night may be associated with increased wakefulness as well as REM sleep rebound. Any improvement in sleep seen early in the night is typically lost during the latter portion of the sleep period. Alcohol can decrease muscle tone in the upper airway and increase the likelihood of both snoring and obstructive sleep apnea; this effect is more pronounced in men than in women. Sleep deprivation potentiates the sedative effects of alcohol, leading to greater impairment than what is seen if one is well rested.

129. Answer: B

EDUCATIONAL OBJECTIVE: Understand the chronic changes in sleep that persist during abstinence from alcohol use.

EXPLANATION: The sleep of alcoholics may be disturbed for months to years after discontinuing alcohol. Many alcoholics feel that alcohol may help them to fall asleep, and complaint of insomnia is a predictor of relapse within a year. Concern with using benzodiazepines in recovering alcoholics is related to the potential for abuse and not loss of efficacy. Polysomnographic studies of sober alcoholics, up to a year after sobriety, continue to show low levels of stage N3 sleep. A shortened REM latency might suggest an ongoing depressive illness, but the former alone does not suggest an ongoing substance abuse.

References:

1. Conroy DA, Todd Arnedt J, Brower KJ, et al. Perception of sleep in recovering alcohol-dependent patients with insomnia: relationship with future drinking. *Alcohol Clin Exp Res.* 2006; 30(12):1992–1999.
2. Drummond SPA, Gillin JC, Smith TL, et al. The sleep of abstinent pure primary alcoholic patients: natural course and relationship to relapse. *Alcohol Clin Exp Res.* 1998; 22:1796–1802.

130. Answer: D

EDUCATIONAL OBJECTIVE: Describe the effects of medications on sleep.

EXPLANATION: During an interview, the patient acknowledges taking desipramine but has stopped taking the medication 1 week before the overnight polysomnographic study. The shortened REM latency and daytime sleepiness could suggest narcolepsy but the patient denies ancillary symptoms of narcolepsy. In addition, the very high REM percentage (as compared to 20% to 25% in normal individuals) is suggestive of REM sleep rebound seen following the discontinuation of an REM-suppressing agent, such as desipramine. A short REM latency is also suggestive of a depressive illness, but the high REM percentage is not consistent with this disorder.

131. Answer: B

EDUCATIONAL OBJECTIVE: Describe the effects of bright light exposure and melatonin administration on the endogenous circadian sleep–wake rhythm.

EXPLANATION: The phase response curve (PRC) illustrates that bright light given after the minimum body temperature will cause a phase advance of the circadian sleep–wake rhythm. The patient has a delayed sleep phase relative to the needs of his academic schedules, and therefore we want to phase advance his rhythms. Bright light applied soon after his minimum body temperature should have a phase-advancing effect. Minimum core body temperature generally occurs about 2 hours prior to habitual waking. Melatonin has a PRC that is opposite to that of light exposure (i.e., exogenous melatonin given in the early evening should cause a phase advance).

132. Answer: C

EDUCATIONAL OBJECTIVE: Understanding monitoring techniques and circadian rhythms.

EXPLANATION: The constant routine protocol is a monitoring technique to help determine the current phase of circadian rhythm or to see changes in circadian rhythms caused by some manipulation. Circadian rhythms can be influenced by a number of factors including light exposure, activity, eating, and even sleeping. The constant routine protocol requires the subjects to remain in a semirecumbent posture for 24 to 48 hours, and sometimes they are kept awake. The subjects are also kept in dim light and in temporal isolation. Food and liquid are provided in 24 equally divided portions. During the study, salivary melatonin levels and core body temperature may be monitored. This is a technically difficult and arduous procedure but can provide accurate estimates of the subjects circadian rhythm while limiting the factors that can influence the rhythm.

Reference:

Herman JH. Chronobiologic monitoring techniques. In: Kryger MH, Roth T, Dement WC, eds. *Principles and Practice of Sleep Medicine.* 4th ed. Philadelphia, Pa: Elsevier; 2005: 1468–1474.

133. Answer: B

EDUCATIONAL OBJECTIVE: Describe the pathophysiology of restless legs syndrome (RLS).

EXPLANATION: Iron is a cofactor for tyrosine hydoxylase, the rate-limiting enzyme in dopamine synthesis. RLS responds to dopaminergic agonists and is made worse by dopamine antagonists, supporting the hypothesis that central dopamine levels may be involved in the disorder. An association between RLS and iron deficiency anemia has been described. Magnetic resonance imaging (MRI) and autopsy studies have shown a number of iron-related abnormalities in the substantia nigra patients with RLS. Since iron is necessary for the synthesis of dopamine, low iron levels can lead to decreased dopamine synthesis in the substantia nigra.

134. Answer: C

EDUCATIONAL OBJECTIVE: Understand the processes that synchronize circadian rhythms.

EXPLANATION: Recently, nonrod, noncone photoreceptors in the ganglion cells of the retina have been identified which are especially important for entraining effects of light. These nonvisual circadian photoreceptors are most sensitive to blue wavelength light. Therefore, blue light exposure may be the most efficient wavelength to shift the circadian sleep–wake rhythm and suppress melatonin. Rods and cones can also influence the circadian response to light. Nonphotic zeitgebers, such as scheduled sleep time and regular meal times, can have an influence on circadian rhythms but their effects are relatively weaker compared to the light–dark cycle. Generally, light intensity of at least 100 lux is necessary to shift rhythms; in individuals living in low-light conditions, significant circadian shifts can occur with light intensities of 50 to 600 lux.

References:

1. Zeitzer JM, Dijk DJ, Kronauer R, et al. Sensitivity of the human circadian pacemaker to nocturnal light: melatonin phase resetting and suppression. *J Physiol.* 2000; 526(Pt 3): 695–702.
2. Berson DM, Dunn FA, Takao M. Phototransduction by retinal ganglion cells that set the circadian clock. *Science.* 2002; 295:1070–1073.
3. Sack RL, Auckley D, Auger R, et al. Circadian rhythm sleep disorders: Part I, Basic principles, shift work and jet lag disorders. An American Academy of Sleep Medicine Review. *Sleep.* 2007; 30(11):1460–1483.

135. Answer: C

EDUCATIONAL OBJECTIVE: Understand the changes in sleep in women during the menstrual cycle.

EXPLANATION: Despite frequent sleep complaints during the premenstrual period, studies have failed to find substantial objective changes in sleep across the menstrual cycle notwithstanding a blunting of the nocturnal drop in core body temperature. Polysomnographic studies have found relatively stable sleep-onset latency and sleep efficiency at different phases of the menstrual cycle. The most consistent findings have been a shortening of REM latency and a slight decrease in REM sleep that may be related to changes in body temperature during the luteal phase. Women taking oral contraceptives show an increase in core body temperature similar to that in the luteal phase. Core body temperature remains elevated throughout the 7-day placebo period of the oral contraceptive pack.

References:

1. Manber R, Armitage R. Sex steroids and sleep: a review. *Sleep.* 2000; 23:145–149.
2. Armitage R, Baker FC, Parry BL. The menstrual cycle and circadian rhythms. In: Kryger M, Roth T, Dement WC, eds. *Principles and Practice of Sleep Medicine.* 4th ed. Philadelphia, Pa: Elsevier Saunders; 2005:1266–1277.

136. Answer: A

EDUCATIONAL OBJECTIVE: Describe the clinical features of jet lag.

EXPLANATION: The type and severity of sleep disturbance associated with jet lag depends on the number of time zones crossed and the direction of travel. Studies of transatlantic flights showed convincingly that westward flight had fewer jet lag effects than did eastward flight. It has been estimated that each postflight day following an eastward flight allows 60 minutes of recovery, whereas following westward flight, each postflight day allows 90 minutes of recovery. Therefore, one can adapt to the new time zone more rapidly following westward flight.

When traveling in an eastward direction, adhering to the home bedtime in the new time zone causes a phase shift in that the bedtime now occurs at a physiologic time earlier than home bedtime. The bedtime would then correspond to a time when the temperature rhythm is still rising and the individual will have more difficulty falling asleep, and there may be more wakefulness early in the night as this time typically corresponds to wakefulness in the home environment.

Travel in a westward direction would have sleep occurring past the falling temperature phase and sleep onset is typically easy and there may be an increase in N3 sleep with an increase in REM sleep on subsequent nights. Awakenings may increase toward the end of the night as this time typically corresponds to daytime in the home time zone.

While the number of time zones crossed certainly has a bearing on the time to adapt to the new time zone, as previously noted, the direction of travel also has a significant influence.

Many studies have demonstrated that countermeasures such as exposure to bright light, use of dark goggles, appropriately timed use of melatonin, and hypnotic medication can have a positive effect on adapting to the new time zone.

References:

1. Sack RL, Auckley D, Auger R, et al. Circadian rhythm sleep disorders: Part I, Basic principles, shift work and jet lag disorders. An American Academy of Sleep Medicine Review. *Sleep.* 2007; 30(11):1460–1483.
2. Arendt J, Stone B, Skene DJ. Sleep disruption in jet lag and other circadian rhythm-related disorders. In: Kryger M, Roth T, Dement WC, eds. *Principles and Practice of Sleep Medicine.* 4th ed. Philadelphia, Pa: Elsevier Saunders; 2005:659–672.
3. Monk TH. Jet lag. In: Lee-Chiong T, ed. *Sleep: A Comprehensive Handbook.* Hoboken, NJ: John Wiley and Sons; 2006:389–393.

137. Answer: B

EDUCATIONAL OBJECTIVE: Describe the performance of multiple sleep latency test (MSLT).

EXPLANATION: In the MSLT clinical protocol, the test is terminated after 20 minutes if no sleep occurs. However, once sleep is identified (i.e., 30 seconds of any sleep stage), the test is allowed to continue for another 15 minutes. If a subject falls asleep within the first epoch of lights out, the shortest a test could be would be 15 minutes. If the subject did not fall asleep until the last epoch at 20 minutes, the test would then be extended an additional 15 minutes giving a maximum duration of 35 minutes.

138. Answer: D

EDUCATIONAL OBJECTIVE: Learn how to evaluate a person presenting with complaints of insomnia.

EXPLANATION: While this gentleman certainly has a number of sleep hygiene issues, these factors alone are usually not the primary cause of the insomnia. Sleep hygiene therapy is usually used in conjunction with other therapies but as a single therapy is not reliably effective in treating insomnia.

Relaxation-based therapies may be considered, as this patient reports being "high strung" but he does not suffer from a specific anxiety disorder. The goal of relaxation therapy is to reduce the level of arousal at bedtime or during arousals from sleep. Relaxation therapy can be effective but is not as effective as sleep restriction therapy.

Stimulus control therapy and sleep restriction therapy are the most commonly used and most effective individual therapies for insomnia. Either therapy could be considered for this subject. The goal of stimulus control therapy is to break the negative associations between presleep rituals and the bedroom environment; these associations can become stimuli for arousal and apprehension rather than sleep. There is, however, no compelling evidence that this patient has developed negative associations related to the bedroom environment. He does not sleep any better in different environments and he felt his sleep in the sleep laboratory was similar to an average night at home.

Sleep restriction therapy is probably the best monotherapy for this patient. He is spending about 11 hours in bed each night, but even under the best of circumstances, he may only get 8 hours of sleep. He reports that he will eventually sleep well after several nights of poor sleep. Sleep restriction therapy attempts to systematically sleep deprive the individual, thus increasing sleep homeostasis and resulting in a more rapid sleep onset as well as decreasing the number and duration of awakenings.

This patient could also have a circadian rhythm sleep disturbance of the delayed sleep phase type. He does not usually fall asleep until 1:00 a.m. and awakens spontaneously at 8:00 a.m. With sleep restriction therapy, the patient is limited to 6 hours in bed by delaying bedtime until 2:00 a.m. and assuring that he is up no later than 8:00 a.m. This will produce a stage 4 sleep deprivation. This technique should increase sleep homeostasis and realign his sleep cycle with his circadian sleep–wake rhythm.

Reference:

Lichstein KL, Riedel BW, Wilson NM, et al. Relaxation and sleep compression for late-life insomnia: a placebo controlled trial. *J Consult Clin Psychol.* 2001; 69:227–239.

139. Answer: A

EDUCATIONAL OBJECTIVE: Learn how menopause affects sleep in women.

EXPLANATION: Apart from the sleep disturbance caused by hot flashes, objective polysomnographic studies examining sleep during menopause have failed to find any substantial changes in sleep quality that would account for the subjective complaint. The changes that occur during sleep may be caused by aging itself rather than a direct consequence of hormonal changes. Hot flashes clearly disrupt sleep and may persist for years or even decades following the last menstrual period. Hormone replacement therapy is the best treatment for hot flashes, and in women with frequent disruption of sleep due to hot flashes, it seems to help increase sleep efficiency, decrease sleep-onset latency, and increase REM sleep. However, in women with mild or infrequent hot flashes, hormone replacement therapy does not have any substantial effect on sleep quality.

References:

1. Young T, Rabago D, Zgierska A, et al. Objective and subjective sleep quality in premenopausal, perimenopausal, and post menopausal women in the Wisconsin Sleep Cohort Study. *Sleep.* 2003; 26:667–672.
2. Moe KE. Menopause. In: Kryger M, Roth T, Dement WC, eds. *Principles and Practice of Sleep Medicine.* 4th ed. Philadelphia, Pa: Elsevier Saunders; 2005:1287–1296.

140. Answer: A

EDUCATIONAL OBJECTIVE: Describe the activation-synthesis theory of dreaming.

EXPLANATION: Activation-synthesis theory ascribes dreaming to brain activation during sleep. As it is in waking, the source of the activation is the reticular formation, but the chemical mode of activation is distinctly different. Noradrenergic and serotonergic systems modulate the activated brain during wakefulness but not in REM sleep dreaming. Without the effects of norepinephrine and serotonin, certain brain structures, such as the cerebral cortex and hippocampus, cannot function as they do during wakefulness; thus, they are not oriented or logical and, as a result, create odd and remote associations, making dreams inherently bizarre.

Reference:

Hobson JA. *The Dream Drugstore.* Cambridge, Mass: The MIT Press; 2001:70–71.

141. Answer: C

EDUCATIONAL OBJECTIVE: Describe changes in the thermoregulation that occur during sleep before bedtime.

EXPLANATION: Body heating, either passively or through exercise, increases stage N3 sleep but has no effect on REM sleep. Total sleep time is greatest at thermoneutrality and decreases as the temperature rises or falls outside this zone. REM sleep appears to be more sensitive than NREM sleep to the temperature changes.

Reference:

Heller HC. Temperature, thermoregulation, and sleep. In: Kryger M, Roth T, Dement WC, eds. *Principles and Practice of Sleep Medicine.* 4th ed. Philadelphia, Pa: Elsevier Saunders; 2005:292–304.

142. Answer: D

EDUCATIONAL OBJECTIVE: Understand the high prevalence of chronic insufficient sleep as a cause of excessive daytime sleepiness.

EXPLANATION: The patient is not sleeping enough each night. The most common cause of excessive daytime sleepiness in the United States is chronic insufficient sleep syndrome. On the basis of self-reports, the prevalence of insufficient sleep is estimated to be 20% of the population. This is often attributed to a lack of opportunity for sleep. The average sleep need is 8 hours a night. The patient does not have a circadian rhythm disorder that could be managed with melatonin and light therapy. His caffeine use is not affecting his ability to fall asleep at night.

References:

1. Hublin C, Kaprio J, Partinin M, et al. Insufficient sleep—a population-based study in adults. *Sleep.* 2001; 24(4):392–400.
2. Groeger JA, Zijlstra FR, Dijk DJ. Sleep quantity, sleep difficulties and their perceived consequences in a representative sample of some 2000 British adults. *J Sleep Res.* 2004; 13(4): 359–371.

143. Answer: C

EDUCATIONAL OBJECTIVE: Understand the strong association between obstructive sleep apnea (OSA) and hypertension.

EXPLANATION: OSA is associated with the development of hypertension. One proposed mechanism by which OSA gives rise to hypertension is chronic stimulation of the sympathetic nervous system with increased catecholamine levels. By monitoring sympathetic nerve activity, respiration, and intra-arterial blood pressure, it has been documented that an increase in sympathetic nerve activity occurs during an episode of obstructive apnea, with a surge in blood pressure occurring at the termination of the apnea. This surge in blood pressure resolves with positive airway pressure therapy.

Reference:

Somers VK, Dyken ME, Clary MP, et al. Sympathetic neural mechanisms in obstructive sleep apnea. *J Clin Invest.* 1995; 96(4):1897–1904.

144. Answer: B

EDUCATIONAL OBJECTIVE: Understand that many patients with obstructive sleep apnea (OSA) may not have complaints of excessive daytime sleepiness.

EXPLANATION: In the Sleep Heart Health Study, the responses on sleepiness questionnaires from individuals with moderate to severe OSA with an apnea–hypopnea index (AHI) ≥15 were evaluated. "Sleepy" was defined as an Epworth Sleepiness Score of greater than 10 or a response of "often" to feeling sleepy or not well rested. Forty-six percent of patients with moderate to severe OSA reported sleepiness, whereas the majority did not. Other potential contributors to subjective sense of sleepiness in patients with sleep-disordered breathing include insomnia, partial sleep deprivation, respiratory disease, and periodic limb movements.

Reference:

Kapur VK, Baldwin CM, Resnick HE, et al. Sleepiness in patients with moderate to severe sleep-disordered breathing. *Sleep.* 2005; 28(4):472–477.

145. Answer: C

EDUCATIONAL OBJECTIVE: Understand that low-intensity monochromatic light in the 460-nm wavelength range has been shown to effectively suppress human melatonin levels.

EXPLANATION: Polychromatic (white) light with an illuminance of 10,000 lux has been recommended as phototherapy to reset the circadian pacemaker. However, recent literature supports the use of low-intensity monochromatic light in the blue range of 460 nm. This short wavelength of light has been shown to suppress human melatonin levels more effectively than 550-nm monochromatic light.

Reference:

Lockley SW, Brainard GC, Czeisler CA. High sensitivity of the human circadian melatonin rhythm to resetting by short wavelength light. *J Clin Endocrinol Metab.* 2003; 88(9):4502–4505.

146. Answer: D

EDUCATIONAL OBJECTIVE: Recognize hypnic jerks on polysomnography.

EXPLANATION: Hypnic jerks (or sleep starts) are sudden and brief contractions of the body occurring at sleep onset. They may be associated with a sensation of falling, dreaming, or hallucinations. They are common with a prevalence of up to 60% to 70% in people. Although generally benign, they can contribute to sleep-onset insomnia. Hypnic jerks are exacerbated by excessive stimulant use, intense physical activity, and emotional stress. Therapy includes treating underlying causes, such as decreasing stimulant use. If necessary, benzodiazepines can be used successfully as a treatment.

Reference:

American Academy of Sleep Medicine. *International Classification of Sleep Disorders: Diagnostic and Coding Manual.* 2nd ed. Westchester, Ill: American Academy of Sleep Medicine; 2005:208–210.

147. Answer: A

EDUCATIONAL OBJECTIVE: Understand how the first-generation antihistamines affect sleep.

EXPLANATION: First-generation antihistamines, such as diphenhydramine, are commonly used as over-the-counter sleep aids. They have more central nervous system effects than later generation antihistamines and, therefore, are more sedating. They induce sedation via central antihistaminergic mechanisms. Histaminergic receptors in the tuberomammillary nuclei and surrounding posterior hypothalamus are involved in arousal. They also possess muscarinic anticholinergic effects. Because acetylcholine is involved in REM sleep generation, REM sleep is reduced because of their anticholinergic effects.

Reference:

Kryger MH, Roth T, Dement WC, eds. *Principles and Practice of Sleep Medicine.* 4th ed. Philadelphia, Pa: Elsevier; 2005:462, 508.

148. Answer: D

EDUCATIONAL OBJECTIVE: Understand that children often present with hyperactivity or behavioral issues rather than excessive sleepiness as a manifestation of sleep-disordered breathing.

EXPLANATION: Attention deficit hyperactivity disorder (ADHD) has been associated with sleep disorders including sleep-disordered breathing and periodic limb movement disorder. The complaint of inattention, hyperactivity, or aggressive behavior may be more common than sleepiness. A complete sleep history followed by nocturnal polysomnography would assist in making the diagnosis of an underlying sleep disorder. If sleep-disordered breathing is detected, treatment with adenotonsillectomy should be considered. Overall, the literature suggests that treating sleep-disordered breathing improves the underlying ADHD.

References:

1. Chervin RD, Dillon JE, Bassetti C, et al. Symptoms of sleep disorders, inattention, and hyperactivity in children. *Sleep.* 1997; 20(12):1185–1192.
2. Huang YS, Guilleminault C, Li HY, et al. Attention-deficit/hyperactivity disorder with obstructive sleep apnea: a treatment outcome study. *Sleep Med.* 2007; 8(1):18–30.

149. Answer: D

EDUCATIONAL OBJECTIVE: Understand the key features of pseudo-spindles.

EXPLANATION: Pseudo-spindles may be observed in patients taking benzodiazepines. An increase in apparent spindle activity on the sleep electroencephalogram in these patients often results in an increase in scoring of stage N2 sleep. The frequencies of pseudo-spindles are slightly higher than the usual beta (12 to 14 Hz) frequency of sleep spindles.

Reference:

Berry RB. *Sleep Medicine Pearls.* 2nd ed. Philadelphia, Pa: Hanley and Belfus; 2002: 4–5.

150. Answer: A

EDUCATIONAL OBJECTIVE: Understand the effects of high altitude on sleep-related breathing disorders.

EXPLANATION: A significant increase in altitude tends to elicit the development of central apneas. This may be due, in part, to a decrease in arterial Pco_2. An increase in central apneas as well as improvement in obstructive apneas at high altitude have been shown using simulation with isobaric hypoxia. Conversely, descent from altitude is associated with a decrease in the apnea–hypopnea index mainly due to a reduction in hypopneas and central apneas. The greater frequency of central apneas at higher elevations is felt to be due to decreased partial pressures of oxygen compared to lower altitudes. For hypopneas, it is possible that a greater drop in oxygen saturation at higher altitude provides a ≥4% oxygen desaturation, which is necessary to define a hypopnea.

References:

1. Burgess KR, Johnson PL, Edwards N. Central and obstructive sleep apnea during ascent to high altitude. *Respirology.* 2004; 9(2):222–229.
2. Burgess KR, Copper J, Rice A, et al. Effect of simulated altitude during sleep on moderate-severity OSA. *Respirology.* 2006; 11(1):62–69.
3. Patz D, Spoon M, Corbin R, et al. The effect of altitude descent of obstructive sleep apnea. *Chest.* 2006; 130(6):1744–1750.

151. Answer: B

EDUCATIONAL OBJECTIVE: Understand the effectiveness of adenotonsillectomy as treatment of obstructive sleep apnea in children.

EXPLANATION: Unlike adults, adenotonsillectomy has been shown to be effective in treating obstructive sleep apnea in most children. After adenotonsillectomy, not only are there improvements in respiratory events, but improvements in behavior, quality of life, and growth have also been noted.

References:

1. Tal A, Bar A, Leiberman A, et al. Sleep characteristics following adenotonsillectomy in children with obstructive sleep apnea syndrome. *Chest.* 2003; 124(3):948–953.
2. Won CH, Li KK, Guilleminault C. Surgical treatment of obstructive sleep apnea: upper airway and maxillomandibular surgery. *Proc Am Thor Soc.* 2008; 5(2):193–199.

152. Answer: B

EDUCATIONAL OBJECTIVE: Understand the effects of different positions and sleep stages on Cheyne–Stokes respiration.

EXPLANATION: This 5-minute polysomnographic tracing demonstrates the typical pattern seen with Cheyne–Stokes respiration, namely, a crescendo–decrescendo respiratory pattern with periods of hyperventilation and hypoventilation. Cheyne–Stokes respiration tends to be more prominent in the supine position. Commonly seen during NREM sleep, the respiratory pattern normalizes during REM sleep.

References:

1. Sahlin C, Svanborg E, Stenlund H, et al. Cheyne–Stokes respiration and supine dependency. *Eur Respir J.* 2005; 25(5):829–833.
2. Solin P, Roebuck T, Swieca J, et al. Effects of cardiac dysfunction on non-hypercapnic central sleep apnea. *Chest.* 1998;113(1):104–110.

153. Answer: B

EDUCATIONAL OBJECTIVE: Recognize the association between enuresis and sleep-disordered breathing.

EXPLANATION: The prevalence of nocturnal enuresis is higher in children with obstructive sleep apnea (OSA), defined as apnea–hypopnea index (AHI) ≥ 1 versus children with AHI < 1. Resolution of enuresis has occurred in some children treated for sleep-disordered breathing. Also, adult nocturnal enuresis has been described as an unusual presentation of OSA. As in children, resolution of enuresis with treatment of OSA has also been reported.

References:

1. Brooks LJ, Topol HI. Enuresis in children with sleep apnea. *J Pediatr.* 2003; 142(5):515–518.
2. Kramer NR, Bonitati AE, Millman RP. Enuresis and obstructive sleep apnea in adults. *Chest.* 1998; 114(2):634–637.

154. Answer: D

EDUCATIONAL OBJECTIVE: Recognize the effects of nicotine on sleep.

EXPLANATION: Increased sleep fragmentation is noted in smokers versus nonsmokers. Increased sleep latency and arousals have been reported. Withdrawal symptoms include an increase in nocturnal arousals as well as an increase in daytime sleepiness.

Reference:

Kryger MH, Roth T, Dement WC, eds. *Principles and Practice of Sleep Medicine.* 4th ed. Philadelphia, Pa: Elsevier; 2005: 1352.

155. Answer: C

EDUCATIONAL OBJECTIVE: Recognize modalities that have been shown to improve compliance to positive airway pressure therapy.

EXPLANATION: Bi-level positive airway pressure (BPAP) has not been shown to improve compliance in unselected patients with obstructive sleep apnea. However, there are reports of improved compliance with BPAP in selected patients participating in a stepwise approach to compliance improvement. The benefit of automatic positive airway pressure (autoPAP) on compliance has also not been conclusively demonstrated. Flexible positive airway pressure therapy may improve therapy compliance in some patients. Heated humidity has been shown to improve CPAP compliance, likely as a result of improved upper airway symptoms.

References:

1. Reeves-Hoche MK, Hudgel DW, Meck R, et al. Continuous versus bi-level positive airway pressure for obstructive sleep apnea. *Am J Respir Crit Care Med.* 1995; 151(2 Pt 1): 443–449.
2. Ballard RD, Gay PC, Strollo PJ. Interventions to improve compliance in sleep apnea patients previously non-compliant with continuous positive airway pressure. *J Clin Sleep Med.* 2007; 3(7):706–712.
3. Berry RB, Parish JM, Hartse KM. The use of auto-titrating continuous positive airway pressure for treatment of adult obstructive sleep apnea. An American Academy of Sleep Medicine Review. *Sleep.* 2002; 25(2):148–173.
4. Aloia MS, Stanchina M, Arnedt JT, et al. Treatment adherence and outcomes in flexible vs standard continuous positive airway pressure therapy. *Chest.* 2005; 127(6):2085–2093.

5. Massie CA, Hart RW, Peralez K, et al. Effects of humidification on nasal symptoms and compliance in sleep apnea patients using continuous positive airway pressure. *Chest.* 1999; 116(2):403–408.

156. Answer: D

EDUCATIONAL OBJECTIVE: Recognize electrocardiogram (ECG) artifact in the electroencephalogram.

EXPLANATION: This electroencephalogram nicely demonstrates an ECG artifact. The spikes correspond to each QRS wave from the ECG signal. It should not be confused with epileptiform activity.

157. Answer: B

EDUCATIONAL OBJECTIVE: Understand the effects of renal failure on sleep apnea syndromes.

EXPLANATION: Sleep disorders are common in chronic renal failure patients, many of whom have sleep-related breathing disorders. Patients tend to be hypocapnic due to underlying metabolic acidosis from their renal disease that affects nocturnal ventilation. Both renal transplantation and conversion from conventional to nocturnal hemodialysis have been shown to decrease central and obstructive apneas in this population.

Reference:

Hanly PJ, Pierratos A. Improvement of sleep apnea in patients with chronic renal failure who undergo nocturnal hemodialysis. *N Engl J Med.* 2001; 344(2):102–107.

158. Answer: A

EDUCATIONAL OBJECTIVE: Understand the pharmacologic features of modafinil.

EXPLANATION: Modafinil, a wake-promoting agent, is cleared hepatically via multiple pathways that include CYP3A4. It may induce the hepatic cytochrome p450 system resulting in the increased metabolism and decreased effectiveness of oral contraceptives. Indications for use include treatment of excessive daytime sleepiness in narcolepsy, shift work sleep disorder, or as an adjunct to continuous positive airway pressure (CPAP) therapy in obstructive sleep apnea. It is not effective in treating cataplexy associated with narcolepsy. As with other stimulants, a concern for long-term cardiovascular risk exists. Its effective half-life is 15 hours with a time to peak serum concentration of 2 to 4 hours.

Reference:

FDA Approved Labeling Text for NDA 20-717/S-005 & S-008. Approved January 23, 2004. Cephalon, Inc.: Patient Information Leaflet. Retrieved October 13, 2008, from http://www.fda.gov/Cder/foi/label/2004/20717se1-008_provigil_lbl.pdf.

159. Answer: C

EDUCATIONAL OBJECTIVE: Understand the relationship between polycystic ovarian syndrome (PCOS) and obstructive sleep apnea (OSA).

EXPLANATION: PCOS is a common endocrine disorder seen in women of reproductive age. Generally, there is an increase in androgenic hormones, anovulation, and insulin resistance. There is an increased prevalence of OSA in women with PCOS versus women without PCOS, even after accounting for differences in the body mass index. Differences in plasma and free testosterone levels between

PCOS patients with and without OSA are not felt to be significant. Compared to PCOS patients without OSA, PCOS patients with OSA have been shown to have higher fasting insulin levels and lower glucose-to-insulin ratios consistent with increased insulin resistance.

Reference:

Vgontzas AN, Legro RS, Bixler EO, et al. Polycystic ovary syndrome is associated with obstructive sleep apnea and daytime sleepiness: role of insulin resistance. *J Clin Endocrinol Metab.* 2001; 86(2):517–520.

160. Answer: C

EDUCATIONAL OBJECTIVE: Recognize the artifact that occurs when an electrode becomes loose during electroencephalographic (EEG) monitoring.

EXPLANATION: The EEG in this epoch demonstrates "electrode popping" in which the involved lead is loose and not completely adherent to the skin. This typically appears as an abrupt change in the signal due to a sudden alteration in electrode impedance. If this appearance occurs in more than one channel, looking for the common reference lead in the abnormal channels identifies the culprit electrode.

161. Answer: A

EDUCATIONAL OBJECTIVE: Understand the difference between restless legs syndrome (RLS) and periodic limb movements (PLMs) on polysomnography.

EXPLANATION: Most patients with RLS will have PLM disorder on polysomnography. However, the converse is not true. The prevalence of PLMs on polysomnography is quite high. Patients do not generally require treatment unless they are symptomatic. RLS, on the other hand, is not diagnosed by polysomnography but rather on presenting symptoms.

Reference:

American Academy of Sleep Medicine. *International Classification of Sleep Disorders: Diagnostic and Coding Manual.* 2nd ed. Westchester, Ill: American Academy of Sleep Medicine; 2005:178–186.

162. Answer: B

EDUCATIONAL OBJECTIVE: Understand the effects of gamma hydroxybutyrate (GHB) in narcolepsy.

EXPLANATION: GHB is an endogenous breakdown product of gamma aminobutyric acid (GABA). Sodium oxybate is the exogenously administered form. Much of its effects appear to be via the GHB and GABA-B receptors. It increases slow-wave sleep and decreases nocturnal arousals. In addition, it has been shown to decrease cataplexy. It is currently indicated only for patients with narcolepsy.

Reference:

Mamelak M, Black J, Montplaisir J, et al. A pilot study on the effects of sodium oxybate on sleep architecture and daytime alertness in narcolepsy. *Sleep.* 2004; 27(7):1327–1334.

163. Answer: B

EDUCATIONAL OBJECTIVE: Recognize the effects of acute sleep deprivation on sleep architecture.

EXPLANATION: After acute sleep deprivation, recovery sleep tends to initially demonstrate an increase in stage N3 sleep. Other stages may be decreased due to the increased amount of stage N3 sleep. This is generally followed by a rebound in REM sleep.

References:

1. De Gennaro L, Ferrara M, Bertini M. The relationship between frequency of rapid eye movements in REM sleep and SWS rebound. *J Sleep Res.* 2000; 9(2):155–159.
2. Kryger MH, Roth T, Dement WC, eds. *Principles and Practice of Sleep Medicine.* 4th ed. Philadelphia, Pa: Elsevier; 2005:61–62.

164. Answer: A

EDUCATIONAL OBJECTIVE: Understand how sleep affects seizure threshold.

EXPLANATION: Seizures may be more prominent during sleep. Seizure threshold is lower during NREM sleep with an increase in epileptiform activity compared to REM sleep. These abnormalities are increased by sleep fragmentation. Nocturnal seizures can contribute to daytime sleepiness, in part, due to sleep fragmentation.

Reference:

Mendez M, Radtke RA. Interactions between sleep and epilepsy. *J Clin Neurophysiol.* 2001; 18(2):106–127.

165. Answer: B

EDUCATIONAL OBJECTIVE: Describe the relationship between prolactin secretion and sleep.

EXPLANATION: Prolactin secretion increases following sleep onset, whether the sleep period occurs at night or during the day. There has been some literature supporting the association between a decreasing rate of prolactin secretion and onset of REM sleep. In addition, an association between hyperprolactinemia and increased stage N3 sleep has been described.

References:

1. Spiegel K, Follenius M, Simon C, et al. Prolactin secretion and sleep. *Sleep.* 1994; 17(1):20–27.
2. Frieboes RM, Murck H, Stalla GK, et al. Enhanced slow wave sleep in patients with prolactinoma. *J Clin Endocrinol Metab.* 1998; 83(8):2706–2710.

166. Answer: A

EDUCATIONAL OBJECTIVE: Recognize the prevalence of sleep-disordered breathing.

EXPLANATION: On the basis of prior data from the Wisconsin Sleep Cohort, the estimated prevalence of sleep-disordered breathing was 4% for men between 30 and 60 years old. This was based on an apnea–hypopnea index (AHI) of ≥5 in the setting of excessive daytime sleepiness. On the basis of AHI alone, about a quarter of men had an AHI ≥5. The prevalence of obstructive sleep apnea (OSA) is likely higher than 4%. In addition, the general body mass index in the United States is increasing. In a 2005 "Sleep in America Poll," about 25% of respondents had a high-risk screen for obstructive sleep apnea based on the Berlin Questionnaire.

References:

1. Young T, Palta M, Dempsey J, et al. The occurrence of sleep-disordered breathing among middle-aged adults. *N Engl J Med.* 1993; 328(17):1230–1235.

2. Hiestand DM, Britz P, Goldman M, et al. Prevalence of symptoms and risk of sleep apnea in the US population: results from the national sleep foundation sleep in America 2005 poll. *Chest.* 2006; 130(3):780–786.

167. Answer: C

EDUCATIONAL OBJECTIVE: Understand factors that may predispose to excessive daytime sleepiness (EDS) in patients with Parkinson disease (PD).

EXPLANATION: Dopaminergic agents, such as levodopa and pramipexole, have been reported to be associated with EDS in patients with PD, although the mechanism is not clear. EDS usually occurs in older patients with longer duration of disease, as opposed to younger patients with less severe disease. Dopaminergic medications do not have any known stimulating properties and have not been reported to improve EDS in PD. Several studies have shown that modafinil is effective in treating EDS in patients with PD, and, in general, amphetamines should be avoided in these patients. Obstructive sleep apnea is commonly seen in patients with PD and may be an important cause of EDS.

Reference:

Adler CH, Thorpy MJ. Sleep issues in Parkinson's disease. *Neurology.* 2005; 64:S12–S20.

168. Answer: D

EDUCATIONAL OBJECTIVE: Comprehend that obstructive sleep apnea (OSA) is an independent risk factor for the development of stroke.

EXPLANATION: Several studies have now shown that OSA is a risk factor for stroke independent of other risk factors such as hypertension, hyperlipidemia, atrial fibrillation, and diabetes. The increased risk of stroke in patients with OSA has not been shown to be due to a patent foramen ovale and occurs equally in men and women. OSA is not a function of temporary pharyngeal instability following a stroke, as some have suggested.

Reference:

Yaggi HK, Conacato J, Kernan WN, et al. Obstructive sleep apnea as a risk factor for stroke and death. *N Engl J Med.* 2005; 353:2034–2041.

169. Answer: A

EDUCATIONAL OBJECTIVE: Understand the relationship between REM sleep behavior disorder (RBD) and the neurodegenerative diseases known as synucleopathies.

EXPLANATION: RBD is a parasomnia characterized by vigorous and sometimes violent behavior in association with dreams. RBD has been noted primarily in middle aged to older men and appears to be a strong predictor of the development of neurodegenerative diseases known as synucleopathies. These disorders are Parkinson disease, Lewy body dementia, and multisystem atrophy. They are all characterized by the presence of α-synuclein positive intracellular inclusions. The frequency of RBD is about 33% to 60% in Parkinson disease, 50% to 80% in Lewy body disease, and 80% to 95% in multisystem atrophy. Alzheimer disease is not classified as one of these diseases and no association has been reported between Alzheimer disease and RBD.

Reference:

Boeve BF, Silber MH, Saper CB, et al. Pathophysiology of REM behaviour disorder and relevance to neurodegenerative disease. *Brain.* 2007; 130:2770–2788.

170. Answer: D

EDUCATIONAL OBJECTIVE: Review the role of iron in the evaluation and management of restless legs syndrome (RLS).

EXPLANATION: There is compelling evidence that iron status is important in the pathogenesis and management of RLS. RLS is a common condition and is influenced by iron stores in the body. Iron deficiency anemia can worsen symptoms of RLS and iron replacement therapy can improve them. Reduced brain stores of iron (specifically in the substantia nigra and the putamen) have been demonstrated by special magnetic resonance imaging (MRI) techniques. Calcium metabolism levels are not known to be associated with RLS. The most sensitive laboratory measurement is the serum ferritin level. A serum ferritin level of less than 50 μg/mL is associated with increased severity of RLS, and iron replacement therapy that increases the ferritin level to greater than 50 μg/mL is associated with improvement in symptoms. Serum ferritin level is much more useful than iron level or the total iron binding capacity.

Reference:

Early CJ. Restless legs syndrome. *N Engl J Med.* 2003; 348:2103–2109.

171. Answer: C

EDUCATIONAL OBJECTIVE: Be aware of research demonstrating abnormalities of hypocretin in narcolepsy/cataplexy syndrome.

EXPLANATION: There has been a significant increase in knowledge about the pathophysiology of narcolepsy in the past 8 years. During that time, it was discovered that patients with narcolepsy and cataplexy have markedly reduced levels of hypocretin in the cerebrospinal fluid and a marked reduction in hypocretin neurons in the brain.

172. Answer: D

EDUCATIONAL OBJECTIVE: Gain knowledge of how the physiology of the circadian rhythms is controlled in part by certain genes and the possibility that certain polymorphisms or mutations of genes can be associated with sleep disorders.

EXPLANATION: The *CLOCK* gene is one of several genes that have been identified to have influence on the circadian cycle. Others include the *TIM* (timeless) and *PER* (period) genes among several others. The CLOCK gene and related mRNA are found in many different cells in the body but the gene oscillates with a circadian rhythm only in the suprachiasmatic nucleus (SCN). A polymorphism of the CLOCK gene has been identified in some families with delayed sleep phase syndrome that occurs in an autosomal dominant mode of inheritance.

173. Answer: A

EDUCATIONAL OBJECTIVE: Understand the changes in ventilation that occur during REM sleep.

EXPLANATION: During REM sleep, there is a reduction in ventilatory response, defined as a change in ventilation following a given change in PaO_2 or $PaCO_2$. The slope of this relationship decreases significantly during REM sleep compared to wakefulness and to NREM sleep. This change is due to altered brainstem responsiveness to PaO_2 and $PaCO_2$, increased upper airway resistance, and decreased skeletal muscle activity during REM sleep. The intercostal muscles become paralyzed and become ineffective in respiration, assuming a smaller role generating tidal volume compared to their activity during wakefulness or NREM sleep. There does not appear to be any gender differences in ventilation during REM sleep and women do not have a different response than men.

174. Answer: A

EDUCATIONAL OBJECTIVE: Be aware of which neurotransmitters are wake inducing and which are sleep inducing.

EXPLANATION: Catecholamines, acetylcholine, hypocretin (also known as orexin), and histamine are wake-producing neurotransmitters in humans. In contrast, serotonin, gamma aminobutyric acid (GABA), and adenosine are major sleep-inducing neurotransmitters. These transmitters are associated with neurons that are distributed widely throughout the brainstem and midbrain. Waking is mediated by neurons in the brainstem reticular formation that extends from the medulla to the midbrain. Sleep is also promoted by neurons located in the lower brainstem reticular formation, solitary tract nucleus, hypothalamus, preoptic area, and basal forebrain.

Reference:

Jones BE. Basic mechanisms of sleep–wake states. In: Kryger MH, Roth T, Dement WC, eds. *Principles and Practice of Sleep Medicine.* Philadelphia, Pa: Elsevier; 2005:136–153.

175. Answer: D

EDUCATIONAL OBJECTIVE: Understand the effects of melatonin on circadian rhythms.

EXPLANATION: Melatonin is a naturally occurring hormone that is tightly correlated with the circadian rhythm. It has been referred to as a "darkness hormone" since it is naturally produced at night, is at its highest levels at night, and its duration of secretion is related to the duration of the night. The exact mechanism of action of melatonin is unknown, but it is known to act as a mild sleep inducing agent, or hypnotic. Its effect, however, depends upon the time of day of administration. If administered during the day, it has a mild soporific effect. If administered several hours before sleep, it has the effect of shortening sleep latency and increasing total sleep time. It can also be used to affect the phase of circadian rhythm and its effect depends on when it is administered in relation to the existing circadian rhythm as measured by core body temperature. If melatonin is administered 5 to 13 hours before core body temperature minimum, it will cause phase advance in the circadian rhythm. If it is administered 5 to 8 hours after core body temperature minimum, the effect will be to delay the circadian rhythm. The action of melatonin on circadian rhythms is the exact opposite of bright light. Bright light will delay circadian rhythms if administered before core body temperature minimum, but will advance circadian rhythms if it is administered after core body temperature minimum.

176. Answer: D

EDUCATIONAL OBJECTIVE: Understand the pulmonary and sleep-related abnormalities seen in patients with restrictive chest wall disease such as kyphoscoliosis.

EXPLANATION: Kyphoscoliosis is a vertebral column and chest wall deformity that causes a restrictive pulmonary defect. Pulmonary function tests commonly show a restrictive pattern with reductions in total lung capacity and vital capacity. Forced expiratory volume in one second (FEV_1) is reduced but normalizes when adjusted for the reduction in forced vital capacity (FVC). Patients often have hypoxia, hypercapnia, and chronic respiratory acidosis with compensatory metabolic alkalosis. Sleep is often disturbed in these individuals with hypoxia and marked oxygen desaturation during sleep. Sleep is characterized by a relative increase in arousals, increased levels of stage N1 and N2 sleep, and lower percentages of stage N3 and stage R sleep. There are often marked REM sleep-related desaturations because the intercostal respiratory muscles are already in a mechanically ineffective position at baseline. During REM sleep, muscle atonia is present in the intercostal muscles, leaving the diaphragm as the only muscle active during inspiration. Since the intercostal muscles are passive, the rib cage is pulled in during inspiration, further impairing chest wall action during inspiration. Patients also have frequent obstructive and central apneas during sleep.

The best treatment is noninvasive positive pressure ventilation (NPPV) that improves both sleep quality and blood gas abnormalities. Zolpidem would not be effective for the mechanisms causing abnormal sleep in these individuals. Supplemental oxygen would help attenuate oxygen desaturations observed during sleep and would increase baseline O_2 saturation, but is not as effective in improving sleep as NPPV. Continuous positive airway pressure (CPAP) has not been found to be effective in these patients and may be difficult to tolerate because of the airflow resistance associated with expiratory positive airway pressures.

177. Answer: A

EDUCATIONAL OBJECTIVE: Know the American Academy of Sleep Medicine (AASM) criteria for scoring stage N3 sleep.

EXPLANATION: According to the recently published guidelines by the AASM, stage N3 sleep is scored when 20% or more of an epoch consists of slow-wave activity, irrespective of age. Slow-wave activity is characterized by waves with frequency of 0.5 to 2.0 Hz and peak-to-peak amplitude >75 mV, measured over the frontal region. These criteria differ slightly from the previous criteria of Rechstaffen and Kales where stage 3 sleep was scored when 20% to 50% of an epoch consists of slow or delta waves, and stage 4 sleep consists of slow waves occupying >50% of an epoch. Under the new AASM criteria, no distinction is made between stages 3 and 4 sleep and the two are grouped together as stage N3 sleep.

References:

1. Iber C, Ancoli-Israel S, Chesson A, et al. for the American Academy of Sleep Medicine. *The AASM Manual for the Scoring of Sleep and Associated Events: Rules, Terminology, and Technical Specifications.* 1st ed. Westchester, Ill: American Academy of Sleep Medicine; 2007.
2. Rechtschaffenen A, Kales A. *A Manual of Standardized Terminology, Techniques, and Scoring Systems for Sleep in Human Subjects.* Los Angeles: UCLA; 1968.

178. Answer: C

EDUCATIONAL OBJECTIVE: Understand the neurophysiology responsible for muscle atonia that occurs during REM sleep.

EXPLANATION: Under normal circumstances, all skeletal muscles are paralyzed during REM sleep. Exceptions include the extraocular eye muscles, diaphragm, and sphincter muscles. As a result, there is normally no muscle activity or movements in dreaming during REM sleep. In individuals who suffer from REM sleep behavior disorder (RBD) there is absence of REM-related atonia. Affected individuals appear to act out their dreams and engage in active, and sometimes violent, behaviors during REM sleep. During polysomnography, there is increased muscle tone during REM sleep (referred to as REM sleep without atonia). The finding of REM without atonia supports a diagnosis of RBD. The neurons involved in generating REM sleep are located in the pons. These neurons are cholinergic neurons, and the injections of a cholinergic agent such as carbachol in this area will induce active sleep (similar to REM sleep) in the cat. There is a subset of these neurons that appear to innervate motoneurons that control muscle tone. These inhibitory neurons are responsible for the inhibition of skeletal muscles that occurs during REM sleep. They utilize glycine as a neurotransmitter, which appears responsible for the inhibition of motoneuron activity and skeletal muscle tone during REM sleep.

179. Answer: C

EDUCATIONAL OBJECTIVE: Understand the use of gamma hydroxybutyrate (GHB) in the clinical management of narcolepsy with cataplexy syndrome.

EXPLANATION: GHB is an effective therapy for the treatment of narcolepsy. It is a natural hormone that acts on gamma aminobutyric acid (GABA)-B receptors and inhibits dopamine. GHB increases slow wave and REM sleep and enhances growth hormone release during sleep. GHB has been used in clinical trials to treat patients with narcolepsy. Two randomized placebo-controlled trials demonstrated improvements in both cataplexy and excessive sleepiness. Because of its short half-life, GHB is administered as two doses at night, a first dose at bedtime and a second dose 3 to 4 hours later. Because of concerns about the illegal abuse of the drug, this drug is dispensed under tightly controlled conditions through a single central pharmacy.

GHB is not used and is not FDA approved for use in restless legs syndrome, REM behavior disorder, or delayed sleep phase syndrome.

Reference:

Mignot E. An update on the pharmacotherapy of excessive daytime sleepiness and narcolepsy. *Sleep Med Rev.* 2004; 8(5):333–338.

180. Answer: A

EDUCATIONAL OBJECTIVE: Understand the effect of a low-frequency filter on electroencephalography (EEG).

EXPLANATION: A low-frequency filter set at 5 Hz eliminates all electric signals with a frequency of 5 Hz or less. Signals greater than 5 Hz would pass unchanged through this filter. Sweat artifacts typically have a frequency of less than 1 to 2 Hz and, hence, would be filtered by a low-frequency filter. Filtering out such an artifact will improve the appearance of the EEG and facilitate the scoring of sleep stages. A 60-Hz artifact is filtered out by high-frequency filter rather than a low-frequency filter. A low-frequency filter set at 5 Hz would attenuate signals of 2 to 4 Hz, which is the frequency of slow or delta waves. As a result, identifying stage

N3 sleep would be more difficult. Sleep spindles have a frequency of 12 to 14 Hz and, hence, would not be filtered by a low-frequency filter; thus, scoring of N2 sleep will not be affected.

181. Answer: C

EDUCATIONAL OBJECTIVE: Be aware of the adverse consequences of chronic benzodiazepine use, including rebound insomnia.

EXPLANATION: The use of benzodiazepines for the treatment of insomnia is common. Benzodiazepines are much safer than once commonly prescribed barbiturates which were used earlier for sleep. However, there are significant adverse reactions secondary to benzodiazepines which the clinician should be aware of. Among these is cognitive impairment, which can be quite severe and cause anterograde amnesia, that is, events that occur while the drug is in the system are forgotten later. Another significant side effect is rebound insomnia; after the drug has been taken for a period of time, sleep is much worse than usual when the drug is stopped abruptly. This acute worsening of sleep may lead patients to believe that they cannot sleep without it. As a result, they may end up using the drug chronically. In reality, the worsening of sleep when the drug is stopped will improve over several weeks. Hypnotics have also been associated with an increase of falls resulting in hip fractures in some studies. Tricyclic antidepressant medications often cause drowsiness as a side effect and are, therefore, often used in lower doses as hypnotics. However, tricyclic antidepressants have significant side effects and drug interactions and thus are not desirable to use over the long term. Therefore, the best answer to the question is to advise the patient on sleep hygiene and cognitive behavioral therapy and to taper the dose of the hypnotic over a reasonable period of time.

182. Answer: D

EDUCATIONAL OBJECTIVE: Recognize the unique pharmacologic mechanism of ramelteon.

EXPLANATION: Ramelteon is a unique hypnotic that has a very high affinity for two melatonin receptors, MT 1 and MT 2. It has little effect on the benzodiazepine receptor. As a result, it does not have the same adverse effects as benzodiazepines. It has three to five times greater affinity for the melatonin receptor than melatonin and is 17 times more potent than melatonin at these receptors. It has been shown to improve sleep latency and sleep efficiency. Eszopiclone is a benzodiazepine receptor agonist. Temazepam is a benzodiazepine with an intermediate duration of action. Trazodone is an antidepressant drug that is used as a hypnotic and does not primarily affect the melatonin receptor.

183. Answer: D

EDUCATIONAL OBJECTIVE: Understand the clinical presentation of narcolepsy.

EXPLANATION: Cataplexy is the symptom that is most specific for narcolepsy. It consists of a sudden onset of loss of muscle tone provoked by emotional responses such as laughter, surprise, startle, or anger. It occurs in approximately two thirds of patients with narcolepsy. Cataplexy may primarily involve the neck and head muscles with the head falling forward. It may also involve the arms or legs. If the legs are involved, the knees may tend to buckle causing the patient to fall. Cataplexy is very specific for narcolepsy. It occurs rarely, if at all, in normal individuals. There are some rare neurologic diseases such as Niemann–Pick disease, in which cataplexy can occur, but otherwise, cataplexy is associated exclusively with the presence of cataplexy. The presence of excessive daytime sleepiness plus a definite history of cataplexy is highly sensitive and specific for a diagnosis of narcolepsy. In contrast, hypnagogic hallucinations, which are dream-like images occurring during the transition between wake and sleep, are relatively common in the normal population and are, thus, neither sensitive nor specific for narcolepsy. Restless legs or periodic leg movements in sleep can occur in patients with narcolepsy but are similarly not very sensitive or specific for the disorder. The presence of excessive daytime sleepiness is essential to make a diagnosis of narcolepsy; however excessive daytime sleepiness occurs for a variety of other reasons such as insufficient sleep or obstructive sleep apnea and does not have as high a diagnostic value in diagnosis as cataplexy does.

184. Answer: C

EDUCATIONAL OBJECTIVE: Know which medications are used in the treatment of narcolepsy.

EXPLANATION: Modafinil has been shown to be effective in the treatment of narcolepsy. Pregabalin is used for the indication of certain chronic pain syndromes or in fibromyalgia. Lamictal is an antiseizure agent, whereas, pramipexole is a dopamine receptor agonist. Two randomized controlled studies have shown a positive effect with the use of modafinil in the treatment of excessive sleepiness in patients with narcolepsy. Sodium oxybate has also been introduced as an effective treatment in narcolepsy. It improves both symptoms of excessive sleepiness as well as cataplexy. It is given as an oral solution that must be taken at bedtime and then about 3 or 4 hours later. Sodium oxybate improves the quality of sleep and decreases daytime sleepiness as well as episodes of cataplexy.

185. Answer: D

EDUCATIONAL OBJECTIVE: Understand the differentiating features of a patient complaining of insomnia from a patient who is a short sleeper.

EXPLANATION: The clinical history described is fairly typical for a diagnosis of a "short sleeper." A short sleeper is an individual who presents with concerns about an inability to sleep as long as others and sleeps 5 or fewer hours per night but shows no evidence of daytime sleepiness or impairment. Sleep patterns are not better explained by another disorder. The short sleeper is different from the individual with insomnia or behaviorally induced insufficient sleep by the absence of any complaints of daytime sleepiness, fatigue, or other impairments attributable to insufficient sleep at night.

This individual is able to function well during the daytime on less than 8 hours of sleep. He has no complaints of excessive sleepiness or excessive fatigue. He is a highly productive individual, has achieved a high level of education, and works well in a job that requires alertness and wakefulness. On the basis of this history, polysomnography is not indicated. Since this individual has no troubles with daytime functioning, a hypnotic agent is not indicated and would not have any value. After a careful history, it would be appropriate to assure him that he is a short sleeper and that no further workup is necessary.

186. Answer: A

EDUCATIONAL OBJECTIVE: Know the relationship of the selective serotonin reuptake inhibitor (SSRI) antidepressant medications as a risk factor for development of REM sleep behavior disorder (RBD).

EXPLANATION: SSRIs are associated with the presence of RBD. Paroxetine is an SSRI and has been noted to cause RBD. SSRIs can also cause rapid eye movements during NREM sleep, referred to as "Prozac eyes." Simvastatin, which is an HMG–CoA reductase inhibitor, has not been associated with RBD. Verapamil is a calcium channel blocker. Zolpidem has been associated with some abnormal behaviors during sleep, such as sleep-related eating or driving, but has not been associated with RBD.

187. Answer: C

EDUCATIONAL OBJECTIVE: Review the pathophysiology of obesity hypoventilation syndrome (OHS).

EXPLANATION: In OHS there is evidence of obesity with a body mass index (BMI) generally greater than 35 as well as hypoventilation ($PaCO_2 > 45$ mm Hg). In OHS, there is actually an increase in the mechanical load on the chest wall and lungs that requires a greater work of breathing. Central ventilatory response to hypoxemia and hypercapnia is depressed. The mechanism for this is unknown but is not likely to be due to cytokines associated with obesity. There is a blunting of the effect of leptin in OHS. Leptin is a hormone that suppresses appetite.

There is increased upper airway resistance, compatible with obstructive sleep apnea that is part of the pathophysiology of the OHS. Patients often respond to positive airway pressure (PAP) for therapy.

188. Answer: A

EDUCATIONAL OBJECTIVE: Understand the outcomes data on uvulopalatopharyngoplasty (UPPP) as a treatment for obstructive sleep apnea (OSA).

EXPLANATION: A meta-analysis published in 1996 systematically reviewed all studies related to surgical outcome of UPPP for OSA and found an overall success rate in all patients of approximately 40%. A higher rate of success was noted if the site of obstruction was in the posterior pharynx (e.g., tonsillar obstruction or redundant soft palate). However, if the major site of obstruction was hypopharyngeal or predominantly involving the tongue, which occurs in most patients with OSA, the probability of success was much lower. UPPP shortens the soft palate but has little effect on the tongue base.

There are no specific clinical findings that predict success following UPPP. Cephalometric radiographs do not accurately predict which patients will respond favorably to UPPP. The Müller technique is a forced inspiratory maneuver that produces collapse of the upper airway and is commonly used during flexible laryngoscopic examination with the patient in the upright position. However, findings on the Müller maneuver do not correlate with surgical success.

Reference:

Elshaug AG. Upper airway surgery should not be the first line treatment for obstructive sleep apnea in adults. *BMJ.* 2008; 236:44–45.

189. Answer: B

EDUCATIONAL OBJECTIVE: Understand the relationship of obstructive sleep apnea (OSA) with pulmonary hypertension (PHTN).

EXPLANATION: Most patients with mild OSA do not have PHTN. PHTN is a complication associated with severe cases of OSA. When PHTN is identified in patients with OSA, it is more likely associated with severe oxygen desaturations. Bosentan would not be the first-line therapy for PHTN associated with OSA; rather, continuous positive airway pressure (CPAP) is the preferred therapy. Typically, patients with OSA have mild degrees of PHTN, usually in the range of 30 to 40 mm Hg systolic pulmonary artery pressure. Bosentan is indicated in those patients with idiopathic forms of PHTN or in severe PHTN associated with scleroderma, and clinical studies have shown a benefit in exercise capacity with the use of bosentan and other related medications in these patients.

190. Answer: A

EDUCATIONAL OBJECTIVE: Know the relationship between obstructive sleep apnea (OSA) and the onset of atrial fibrillation.

EXPLANATION: One large study has demonstrated that OSA is an independent predictor for the development of atrial fibrillation independent of other risk factors for the disorder, such as coronary artery disease or congestive heart failure. Like obesity, OSA is also an independent risk for mortality from cardiovascular disease. While ventricular dysrhythmias can be observed in severe OSA, it is also just as common to see atrial arrhythmias, especially atrial fibrillation, in patients with OSA. Atrial fibrillation can develop in patients with OSA even in the absence of severe heart failure or/and the presence of normal ejection fraction.

Reference:

Gami AS, Hodge DO, Herges RM, et al. Obstructive sleep apnea, obesity, and the risk of incident atrial fibrillation. *J Am Coll Cardiol.* 2007; 49:565–571.

191. Answer: A

EDUCATIONAL OBJECTIVE: Be aware that in patients with obstructive sleep apnea (OSA), the highest incidence of sudden cardiac death occurs during the sleep hours between midnight and 6:00 a.m.

EXPLANATION: Sudden death is not a common occurrence in OSA. Normal people generally arouse from sleep when there is airway occlusion. Hence, individuals with OSA do not simply stop breathing and die. Nonetheless, patients with OSA who have significant oxygen desaturation may suffer cardiac dysrhythmias. Thus, patients with a diagnosis of OSA are more likely to sustain sudden cardiac death during the usual sleep hours of midnight to 6:00 a.m., compared to any other 6-hour segment during the day. In contrast, patients without OSA have the highest incidence of sudden cardiac death between the hours of 6:00 a.m. to noon.

Reference:

Gami AS, Howard DE, Olson EJ, et al. Day–night pattern of sudden death in obstructive sleep apnea. *N Engl J Med.* 2005; 352:1206–1214.

192. Answer: B

EDUCATIONAL OBJECTIVE: Review the abnormal patterns of sleep associated with Alzheimer disease (AD).

EXPLANATION: AD is associated with abnormalities in sleep. There is often marked disruption of sleep architecture. REM episodes and REM density are decreased. The phenomenon known as "sundowning" is common in AD and reflects reversal of the usual day–night sleep pattern. Patients may, therefore, sleep during the daytime and are awake and wander during the night. Sundowning is a common indication for admission to long-term care facilities and is the most distressing sleep-related disorder for these individuals. In contrast to Parkinson disease, however, REM sleep behavior disorder is not commonly observed in AD and does not precede the diagnosis of the disorder.

193. Answer: C

EDUCATIONAL OBJECTIVE: Understand the role of bright light therapy in the treatment of seasonal affective disorder (SAD).

EXPLANATION: Patients with SAD may benefit from bright light therapy at an intensity of 10,000 lux for 30 minutes in the morning after awakening; 2,500 lux has also been described, but must be given for at least 2 hours in the morning. (Two hours of therapy would be impractical for most patients.) Bright light of 2,000 lux administered in the late afternoon prior to bedtime is not effective in treating SAD. Administration of 10,000 lux for 2 hours is excessive and unnecessary. While light therapy is generally safe, there is risk of retinal damage if used for prolonged periods of time.

194. Answer: B

EDUCATIONAL OBJECTIVE: Understand the use of sleep diaries in aiding the diagnosis of circadian sleep disorders.

EXPLANATION: The patient gives a history compatible with delayed sleep phase syndrome (DSPS) rather than narcolepsy. She relates a history of staying awake until the early hours of the morning and then desiring sleep until late morning or early afternoon. She has trouble making it to morning classes and has a tendency to fall asleep in them. On weekends, she sleeps until noon or early afternoon. There is no history of cataplexy. The presence of sleep paralysis is not specific for narcolepsy.

DSPS is very common in young adults. A 2-week sleep diary would be very helpful in documenting the sleep–wake patterns. It would not be cost effective to proceed with other tests at this time, such as polysomnography or multiple sleep latency testing. While many patients with narcolepsy carry the HLA DQB1*0602 allele, the latter is also common in the general population and does not have diagnostic value in discriminating narcolepsy from other disorders. Similarly, while there is substantial evidence that hypocretin levels are reduced in the cerebrospinal fluid of patients with narcolepsy, this test is not readily available in most clinical practices, and would not be indicated in the initial evaluation of this patient. As initial evaluation, a good history aided by sleep diaries may be all that is necessary. Careful follow-up is important to monitor response to counseling and specific interventions and to observe for any new symptoms.

195. Answer: D

EDUCATIONAL OBJECTIVE: Understand the changes in ventilatory patterns that occur during NREM sleep compared to wakefulness.

EXPLANATION: As the brain transitions between wakefulness and sleep, there is a temporary instability in respiration caused by a change in responsiveness to PaO_2 and $PaCO_2$. As sleep occurs, $PaCO_2$ increases by 2 to 8 mm Hg, and PaO_2 decreases by about 3 to 10 mm Hg. There is a relative reduction in ventilation rather than hyperventilation. The decrease in ventilation is primarily due to an increase in upper airway resistance rather than bronchoconstriction.

196. Answer: B

EDUCATIONAL OBJECTIVE: Understand the principle underlying stimulus control therapy (SCT).

EXPLANATION: SCT is based on the principle of classical conditioning. The major assumption is that sleep-incompatible behaviors become paired with the sleep environment so that the sleep environment itself becomes a stimulus to arousal rather than to sleep. The bed, bedroom, and even the rituals of getting ready for bed (e.g., putting on nightclothes or teeth brushing) can become paired with arousal. As a result, the approach to bed can be a stimulus to tension and wakefulness, rather than relaxation. The goal of SCT is to reassociate the feeling of sleepiness with the bedroom and to break the negative conditioning. This is accomplished by having the patient spend time in bed only when sleepy or asleep. By pairing sleep with the bed and bedroom, the environment once again becomes a stimulus to sleep.

197. Answer: C

EDUCATIONAL OBJECTIVE: Describe the adverse effects of chronic use of hypnotic medications.

EXPLANATION: Rebound insomnia occurs following discontinuation of hypnotic medications, particularly short-acting benzodiazepines. For one to two nights following drug discontinuation, sleep may actually be worse than baseline levels. Sleep quality usually returns to baseline levels after a few nights. Longer-acting benzodiazepines, such as flurazepam, are less likely to cause rebound insomnia. However, some reports find that rebound insomnia with longer-acting agents occurs several days after discontinuation and may last longer. The non-benzodiazepine benzodiazepine receptor hypnotics, such as zolpidem, are also less likely to be associated with rebound insomnia. Individual differences, duration of medication use, and half-life of the compound may all influence the development of rebound insomnia.

Reference:

Morin CM. *Insomnia: Psychological Assessment and Management.* New York, NY: The Guilford Press; 1993:161.

198. Answer: B

EDUCATIONAL OBJECTIVE: Understand the effects of psychiatric disorders on sleep.

EXPLANATION: As with generalized anxiety disorder (GAD), most patients with panic disorder (PD) have significant sleep complaints. Their subjective complaints are similar to those patients with GAD. The major difference is the presence of panic attacks. PD patients have longer sleep-onset latencies, decreased sleep efficiency, and decreased total sleep time. Patients may have more movement time during sleep.

However, stage N3 sleep is normal, REM sleep latency is normal or increased, and REM density is normal. About 69% of PD patients describe a lifetime prevalence of panic attacks arising from sleep, and about 33% report recurrent sleep panic attacks. If panic attacks are frequent, patients can develop sleep phobia. Panic attacks generally arise out of late N2 or early N3 sleep. Patients with PD can generally differentiate panic attacks from REM/sleep-related anxiety dreams or sleep terrors. Panic attacks typically are not associated with dream content or vivid imagery. Patients have full awakenings from the event, are not confused at the time of the event, and are not amnestic for the events the following day.

Reference:

Mellman TA, Uhde T. Sleep panic attacks: new clinical findings and theoretical implications. *Am J Psychiatry.* 1989; 146:1204–1207.

199. Answer: C

EDUCATIONAL OBJECTIVE: Describe the sleep characteristics of patients with schizophrenia.

EXPLANATION: The most reliable sleep changes found in schizophrenia occur in NREM sleep, particularly deficits of N3 sleep or delta wave (0.5 to 3 Hz) activity. In addition, many studies have failed to find a rebound of N3 sleep following sleep deprivation. There is a great deal of variability in REM sleep measures in schizophrenic patients, and these differences vary over the course of the illness. Many studies have found shortened REM sleep latencies in unmedicated patients but this is not consistently described. In addition, a longitudinal study found changes in the REM sleep measures but not in slow-wave sleep measures. Although still speculative, the deficit of N3 sleep in the first NREM period may allow REM sleep to occur earlier and could be contributing to the shortened REM latency seen in some studies. Dreaming has been likened to a model for psychosis and hallucinations, but studies have failed to find much convincing evidence of an association between REM sleep abnormalities and hallucinations.

References:

1. Monti JM, Monti D. Sleep in schizophrenia patients and the effects of antipsychotic medications. *Sleep Med Rev.* 2004; 8:133–148.
2. Keshavan MS, Reynolds CF, Miewald JM, et al. A longitudinal study of EEG sleep in schizophrenia. *Psychiatry Res.* 1996; 59(3):203–211.
3. Hobson JA. *The Dream Drugstore—Chemically Altered States of Consciousness.* Cambridge, Mass: The MIT Press; 2001:238–241.

200. Answer: C

EDUCATIONAL OBJECTIVE: Understand the biochemistry responsible for sleep and wakefulness.

EXPLANATION: The three main nuclei of the reticular activating system (RAS) are the pedunculopontine nucleus (PPN) containing acetylcholine, the locus coeruleus (LC) containing norepinephrine, and the raphe nucleus (RN) containing serotonin. All three nuclei are very active during wakefulness. During NREM sleep, their activity decreases but PPN is least active during N3 relative to LC and RN. In REM sleep, the activity is reversed; PPN becomes very active and both LC and RN almost cease to fire. These firing patterns are consistent with the cholinergic REM activating (REM-on) cells in the PPN and laterodorsal tegmental nucleus (LDT) and the REM terminating (REM-off) cells in the LC and RN.

201. Answer: B

EDUCATIONAL OBJECTIVE: Describe the neurotransmitters affecting sleep.

EXPLANATION: The tuberomamillary nucleus (TMN) is the primary source of histamine in the central nervous system (CNS). Histamine is excitatory, and blocking histamine can cause sedation and sleepiness. The excitatory orexin neurons from the lateral hypothalamus promote waking largely through activation of the TMN histaminergic neurons. The TMN neurons are tonically active during wakefulness and significantly decrease firing during sleep.

Reference:

Garcia-Rill E, Wallace T, Good C. Neuropharmacology of sleep and wakefulness. In: Lee-Chiong T, ed. *Sleep: A Comprehensive Handbook.* Hoboken, NJ: John Wiley and Sons; 2006: 63–71.

202. Answer: A

EDUCATIONAL OBJECTIVE: Describe the changes in sleep following total sleep deprivation.

EXPLANATION: A series of experiments in a number of species including humans have examined recovery sleep following a period of total sleep deprivation. These experiments have demonstrated the basic necessity of delta sleep (<4 Hz). Delta waves occur mostly during N3 sleep. In these experiments, N3 sleep rebounds most completely, indicating a higher homeostatic demand for this sleep stage. During recovery sleep following total sleep deprivation, only about 30% of sleep lost is regained. However, all of the missed N3 sleep is recovered. About 50% of the missed stage REM is recovered and very little of N1 and N2 sleep are regained.

References:

1. Horne JA. Sleep function, with particular reference to sleep deprivation. *Ann Clin Res.* 1985; 17:199–208.
2. Payne JD, Walker MP. Does delta sleep matter. *Insomnia.* 2008; 10:3–10.

203. Answer: D

EDUCATIONAL OBJECTIVE: Understand the mechanism of action of wake-promoting agents.

EXPLANATION: Modafinil is a novel wake-promoting substance that is chemically unrelated to the amphetamines or other known stimulants. The mechanism of action of modafinil remains unclear. Amphetamine induces release of dopamine and also blocks its reuptake. Modafinil does not appear to work through dopaminergic mechanisms. Drugs that block synthesis of dopamine (αMPT) substantially block the effects of amphetamine. The wake-promoting effects of modafinil are not blocked with αMPT suggesting that the drug may have a novel mechanism of action. Controlled studies in animals show that modafinil activates certain areas of the brain such as the histaminergic tuberomammillary nucleus and hypocretin-containing cells of the lateral hypothalamus. Modafinil may also decrease activity in the gamma aminobutyric acid (GABA)–containing ventrolateral preoptic nucleus (VLPO). There is no evidence that modafinil acts like methylxanthines by antagonism of adenosine. Although these studies provide clues to the brain areas affected by modafinil, its precise mechanism of action remains unknown.

Reference:

Scammell TE, Estabrooke IV, McCarthy MT, et al. Hypothalamic arousal regions are activated during modafinil-induced wakefulness. *J Neurosci.* 2000; 20:8620–8628.

204. Answer: A

EDUCATIONAL OBJECTIVE: Describe the consequences of smoking on sleep.

EXPLANATION: Nicotine is a major component of cigarette smoke and can negatively affect sleep during use and withdrawal. Polysomnographic studies have demonstrated increased sleep latency, increased arousals, and difficulty staying asleep at night in active smokers compared to nonsmokers. Because of the short half-life of the drug (about 2 hours), sensitive individuals may wake up to smoke at night in response to drops in nicotine levels in the brain during sleep. Tobacco smoke can cause nasal and pharyngeal irritation, thus, narrowing the upper airway. Both apnea and snoring are more prevalent in current smokers than in nonsmokers or former smokers. The discontinuation of nicotine in dependent individuals is associated with disturbances of both sleep and alertness. Transdermal nicotine delivery reduces total sleep time and sleep efficiency, decreases REM sleep, and prolongs sleep latency.

References:

1. Wetter DW, Young TB, Bidwell TR, et al. Smoking as a risk factor for sleep-disordered breathing. *Arch Intern Med.* 1994; 154:2219–2224.
2. Shin C, Joo S, Kim J, et al. Prevalence and correlates of habitual snoring in high school students. *Chest.* 2003; 124:1709–1715.
3. Roehrs T, Roth T. Sleep–wakefulness and drugs of abuse. In: Lee-Chiong T, Sateia M, Carskadon M, eds. *Sleep Medicine.* Philadelphia, Pa: Hanley and Belfus; 2002:575–585.

205. Answer: A

EDUCATIONAL OBJECTIVE: Describe the clinical features of Kleine–Levin syndrome.

EXPLANATION: Kleine–Levin syndrome is a rare and poorly understood disorder characterized by recurrent periods of hypersomnia. Episodes can last a few days to weeks at a time. The interval between episodes can be weeks to months. Although a number of other symptoms are thought to be associated with the disorder (i.e., strong adolescent male predominance, hyperphagia, and hypersexuality), these symptoms may be overrated. Between episodes, cognitive function and sleep are normal. Insomnia is not a prominent feature of the disorder, although, while total sleep time increases during an episode, sleep efficiency is decreased. Cataplexy is not a feature of this syndrome.

Reference:

1. Gadoth N, Kesler A, Vainstein G, et al. Clinical and polysomnographic characteristics of 34 patients with Kleine-Levin Syndrome. *J Sleep Res.* 2001; 10:337–341.
2. Shouse MN, Mahowald MW. Epilepsy, sleep, and sleep disorders. In: Kryger MH, Roth T, Dement WC, eds. *Principles and Practice of Sleep Medicine.* 4th ed. Philadelphia, Pa: Elsevier Saunders; 2005:863–878.

206. Answer: D

EDUCATIONAL OBJECTIVE: Understand the mechanisms for nocturia in obstructive sleep apnea (OSA).

EXPLANATION: Nocturia is a common symptom in patients with OSA. Studies have shown that breathing against a closed airway increases the secretion of a potent diuretic, atrial natriuretic peptide. In addition, there is increased intra-abdominal pressure causing a need to urinate and the frequent awakening associated with OSA can lead the mistaken idea that the need to urinate was the cause of the awakening when in fact it was the apneic event. Other factors include the use of diuretic medications, diabetes mellitus, and excessive fluid intake due to a dry mouth sensation from snoring or mouth breathing. Urinary frequency generally decreases once OSA is treated with nasal continuous positive airway pressure (CPAP).

207. Answer: D

EDUCATIONAL OBJECTIVE: Understand treatment approaches for insomnia.

EXPLANATION: The patient has a relevant clinical history of insomnia with psychophysiologic hyperarousal and a past medical history of depression. In addition, there is enough clinical data to suspect sleep-related breathing disorder (SRBD). The patient's postmenopausal status, nocturnal awakenings with perspiration, elevated body mass index (BMI), and upper airway anatomy make it necessary to consider a clinical diagnosis of SRBD. Treatment with hypnotics and no further assessment of a possible diagnosis of SRBD would not be desirable. Cognitive behavioral therapy for insomnia (CBT-I) might be beneficial but delaying identification of SRBD does not represent a desirable management course. A referral for psychiatric consultation is premature, as the patient does not identify symptoms of depression at the time of consultation.

Reference:

Winkelman JW (Chair), et al. American Academy of Sleep Medicine. *Case Book of Sleep Medicine* (ICSD-2). Westchester, Ill: AASM; 2008.

208. Answer: C

EDUCATIONAL OBJECTIVE: Identify circadian rhythm sleep disorders as a cause of chronic insomnia and sleepiness.

EXPLANATION: Eszopiclone is a relatively long-acting hypnotic, which in this case might leave the patient with significant drowsiness in the morning, the time when he is most sleepy. Citalopram is not indicated, as there is no clinical evidence of relevant anxiety in the patient's clinical presentation. Polysomnography is unlikely to provide significant additional information at this junction but might become necessary depending on the patient's clinical progress. The patient should be provided with instructions on stimulus control therapy and be asked to keep a sleep diary to evaluate for a possible diagnosis of circadian rhythm sleep disorder, delayed sleep phase type.

Reference:

Winkelman JW (Chair), et al. American Academy of Sleep Medicine. *Case Book of Sleep Medicine* (ICSD-2). Westchester, Ill: AASM; 2008.

209. Answer: C

EDUCATIONAL OBJECTIVE: Describe the performance and scoring of a multiple sleep latency test (MSLT).

EXPLANATION: Sleep-onset latency should be scored for each nap opportunity of an MSLT. The sleep-onset latency is scored from the initiation of the nap opportunity to the first epoch containing 15 seconds of any stage of sleep.

Reference:

Iber C, Ancoli-Israel S, Chesson A, et al. American Academy of Sleep Medicine. *The AASM Manual for the Scoring of Sleep and Associated Events: Rules, Terminology and Technical Specifications.* 1st ed. Westchester, Ill: AASM; 2007.

210. Answer: C

EDUCATIONAL OBJECTIVE: Describe positive airway pressure therapy for obstructive sleep apnea (OSA).

EXPLANATION: The patient has significant evidence of moderate to severe OSA. While the Epworth Sleepiness Scale (ESS) is not significant, the description of the other relevant clinical findings and the data derived from overnight ambulatory oximetry indicate a likely diagnosis of OSA. Bi-level positive airway pressure (BiPAP) does not offer significant therapeutic advantages in the management of uncomplicated OSA. Otolaryngology consultation is not warranted given that there is no polysomnographic corroboration of the diagnosis and there is no clinical data indicating relevant findings in the examination of the upper airway.

211. Answer: D

EDUCATIONAL OBJECTIVE: Identify clinical features of narcolepsy without cataplexy.

EXPLANATION: The absence of clinical evidence of a psychotic condition precludes the need for continued therapy with quetiapine. Lorazepam is not indicated for the treatment of hypnagogic hallucinations. The clinical diagnosis is consistent with narcolepsy without cataplexy. Ideally, the sleep laboratory assessment should be completed in a drug-free status.

212. Answer: D

EDUCATIONAL OBJECTIVE: Understand issues related to sleepiness among commercial airline pilots.

EXPLANATION: The primary concern of the Federal Aviation Administration (FAA), as it relates to sleep disorders, is to document alertness. Ideally, the patient should have been prescribed a continuous positive airway pressure (CPAP) unit with a compliance monitor to adequately document treatment adherence. The FAA usually requires documentation of a normal maintenance of wakefulness test (MWT) prior to granting medical certification.

213. Answer: C

EDUCATIONAL OBJECTIVE: Describe the management of suspected obstructive sleep apnea (OSA).

EXPLANATION: OSA is a major contributor to daytime drowsiness, which might prove deadly for commercial truck drivers. Furthermore, truck drivers are at a higher risk of OSA. The patient's clinical presentation, with treatment-resistant hypertension, should further increase the suspicion of OSA. A score of 4 on the Epworth Sleepiness Scale (ESS) should not negatively impact the suspicion of OSA in this patient, as an individual might be unaware of their own sleepiness.

214. Answer: A

EDUCATIONAL OBJECTIVE: Understand when to refer a patient with chronic insomnia for sleep medicine consultation.

EXPLANATION: Further understanding of the patient's overall clinical status is necessary to provide adequate advice on how to best manage this patient's sleep problems. The patient's previous experience with other hypnotics should raise concern of possible tolerance to the continued use of benzodiazepines.

215. Answer: B

EDUCATIONAL OBJECTIVE: Describe the clinical features of paradoxical insomnia.

EXPLANATION: Paradoxical insomnia is characterized by a complaint of severe insomnia that occurs without evidence of objective sleep disturbance. The availability of a normal diagnostic polysomnography in conjunction with the patient's estimates of her sleep enables the correct diagnosis.

216. Answer: B

EDUCATIONAL OBJECTIVE: Describe the clinical features of narcolepsy.

EXPLANATION: Cataplexy is recognized as the unique symptom of narcolepsy. Hypnagogic hallucinations and sleep paralysis are also abnormal manifestations of REM sleep but are not considered pathognomonic of the disorder.

217. Answer: B

EDUCATIONAL OBJECTIVE: Describe the clinical features of insufficient sleep syndrome.

EXPLANATION: Sleep offset paralysis may be a manifestation of REM pressure due to behaviorally induced insufficient sleep. The available information suggests a very restricted sleep schedule. The patient's symptoms will likely be reversed by behavioral modification. If symptoms persist, sleep laboratory evaluation would be indicated. Symptomatic therapy is premature at this time. Determination of cerebrospinal fluid (CSF) hypocretin levels does not represent, at the present time, the standard of care in the diagnosis of narcolepsy.

218. Answer: C

EDUCATIONAL OBJECTIVE: Identify medication-induced hypersomnolence.

EXPLANATION: The available information indicates that the patient has remained stable for a number of years. The most prudent action is to determine if discontinuation of clonazepam represents a viable intervention for this patient. Tapering should be slow. If symptoms remain unchanged, sleep laboratory assessment should be considered. Symptomatic treatment of sleepiness is not indicated. The use of an alternative benzodiazepine might be considered but is unlikely to provide a solution to the patient's symptoms.

219. Answer: A

EDUCATIONAL OBJECTIVE: Describe the differential diagnosis of excessive sleepiness.

EXPLANATION: The patient's presentation is entirely consistent with the International Classification of Sleep Disorders (ICSD) criteria for nonorganic hypersomnia. The description of the patient's symptoms is consistent with a depressive episode.

Reference:

American Academy of Sleep Medicine. *International Classification of Sleep Disorders: Diagnostic and Coding Manual.* 2nd ed. Westchester, Ill: AASM; 2005.

220. Answer: D

EDUCATIONAL OBJECTIVE: Describe the features of the different subjective scales for sleepiness.

EXPLANATION: The Stanford Sleepiness Scale is best used in the laboratory among normal volunteers participating in research studies. It consists of seven items. Subjects are asked to select one item that best describes them at the time of the assessment. The Epworth Sleepiness Scale (ESS) and Sleep–Wake Activity Inventory (SWAI)—EDS Scale are indicated for clinical use to determine subjective levels of sleepiness of an individual and were validated against the multiple sleep latency test (MSLT). A score of >10 on the ESS is generally considered clinically significant. A score of ≤40 on the SWAI—EDS Scale is considered indicative of excessive sleepiness.

221. Answer: A

EDUCATIONAL OBJECTIVE: Describe the different assessment tools for circadian and sleep–wake rhythms.

EXPLANATION: The Sleep–Wake Activity Inventory (SWAI) has been used mostly in the assessment of subjective levels of sleepiness–alertness and does not represent an adequate tool in the assessment of circadian rhythm disorders. The measurement of the temperature rhythm and the dim-light melatonin onset represent tools in the measurement of circadian timing. The Horne–Ostberg questionnaire is a useful tool to assess chronotype.

222. Answer: A

EDUCATIONAL OBJECTIVE: Differentiate tonic from phasic REM sleep.

EXPLANATION: The physiologic phenomena occurring during REM sleep are separated into phasic and tonic events. Muscle atonia is considered one of the hallmarks of tonic REM sleep. Autonomic irregularities, rapid eye movements, and ponto-geniculate-occipital (PGO) waves are considered phasic events.

223. Answer: A

EDUCATIONAL OBJECTIVE: Identify the features of ponto-geniculate-occipital (PGO) waves.

EXPLANATION: Gamma aminobutyric acid (GABA)ergic neurons are believed to induce NREM sleep. PGO waves represent the first sign of REM sleep and are considered phasic manifestations of REM sleep. They are generated in the pons, move on to the lateral geniculate nucleus in the hypothalamus, and end in the occipital cortex.

224. Answer: B

EDUCATIONAL OBJECTIVE: Describe the changes in sleep following sleep deprivation.

EXPLANATION: The expected response to sleep deprivation is increased auditory awakening thresholds. Features consistent with increased sleep pressure secondary to sleep deprivation also include an increase in N3 sleep and total sleep time as well as decrease in sleep-onset latency.

225. Answer: A

EDUCATIONAL OBJECTIVE: Define sleep-onset REM (SOREM) period.

EXPLANATION: SOREM is defined as an REM latency of ≤15 minutes on a multiple sleep latency test.

226. Answer: B

EDUCATIONAL OBJECTIVE: Describe the consequences of REM sleep deprivation.

EXPLANATION: One night of selective REM sleep deprivation has been shown to have no significant effect on the multiple sleep latency test (MSLT). In humans, REM sleep deprivation has been successfully used to treat depression. Acute REM sleep deprivation in healthy subjects has also been shown to increase sensitivity to acute pain.

227. Answer: A

EDUCATIONAL OBJECTIVE: Describe the features of pharmacologic tolerance.

EXPLANATION: Symptoms of withdrawal are usually a reflection of physical dependence. A maladaptive pattern of drug use reflects problems of addiction. Tolerance represents a potentially relevant phenomenon in the pharmacologic management of insomnia.

228. Answer: D

EDUCATIONAL OBJECTIVE: Identify indications that can cause REM sleep behavior disorder.

EXPLANATION: Bupropion works by enhancing dopamine and norepinephrine in the brain. It has not been associated with causing abnormal motor behaviors during sleep. The other listed medications affect serotonin, which have been associated with abnormal motor behaviors during sleep.

229. Answer: D

EDUCATIONAL OBJECTIVE: Identify the half-life of the different hypnotic medications.

EXPLANATION: The drug with the longest half-life, 40+ hours, is flurazepam.
Zolpidem: half-life 1.4 to 4.54 hours
Briazolam: half-life 1.5 to 5.5 hours
Eszopiclone: half-life 6 hours
Flurazepam: half-life 2.3-100 hours

230. Answer: A

EDUCATIONAL OBJECTIVE: Describe the polysomnographic features of primary insomnia.

EXPLANATION: The high sleep efficiency is not consistent with polysomnographic evidence of insomnia. A delayed sleep-onset latency and disturbed sleep continuity and architecture are, on the other hand, consistent with polysomnographic evidence of insomnia.

231. Answer: D

EDUCATIONAL OBJECTIVE: Identify the half-lives of the various non-benzodiazepine benzodiazepine receptor agonists.

EXPLANATION: The hypnotic with the shortest half-life (1 hour) is zaleplon. Zolpidem has a half-life of 2.5 hours and eszopiclone has a half-life of 6 hours. Thus, eszopiclone is the most likely hypnotic to cause residual sedation.

232. Answer: D

EDUCATIONAL OBJECTIVE: Describe the different treatment options for obstructive sleep apnea.

EXPLANATION: Continuous positive airway pressure (CPAP) has been shown to be about 75% effective in the reduction of the apnea–hypopnea index (AHI). The uvulopalatopharyngoplasty (UPPP) is successful in 40% to 50% of the cases. The pillar procedure has been found to reduce the AHI by ≤50% in 45% of subjects when compared to 0% in the placebo group. Temporomandibular joint (TMJ) constitutes a contraindication for oral appliance therapy.

Reference:

1. Hoffstein V. Review of oral appliances for treatment of sleep-disordered breathing. *Sleep Breath* 2007; 11:1–22.
2. Friedman M, Lin HC, Gurpinar B, et al. Minimally invasive single-stage multilevel treatment for obstructive sleep apnea/hypopnea syndrome. *Laryngoscope* 207; 117:1859–1863.

233. Answer: C

EDUCATIONAL OBJECTIVE: Understand how to monitor adherence to continuous positive airway pressure (CPAP) therapy.

EXPLANATION: The average number of CPAP sessions per use days is the least critical value, as it only reflects the number of times that the unit is turned on. Ideally, patients with CPAP should use the therapy on 100% of the days. To the extent that the patient skips the use of CPAP more frequently, the difference between the average time used per day (during the total period) and the average use per night (on nights with CPAP utilization) will grow more significant.

234. Answer: A

EDUCATIONAL OBJECTIVE: Describe effective measures for enhancing adherence to positive airway pressure therapy.

EXPLANATION: While there is Federal Drug Administration (FDA) approval for the use of modafinil in the treatment of residual sleepiness among patients with obstructive sleep apnea (OSA), the patient has not achieved a desirable level of therapeutic adherence to continuous positive airway pressure (CPAP). The most important set of actions should be directed at improving CPAP adherence. The use of the humidifier might help the patient improve her tolerance to therapy.

235. Answer: A

EDUCATIONAL OBJECTIVE: Describe the performance of a multiple sleep latency test (MSLT).

EXPLANATION: While short REM latencies were documented on the test, the test was not completed following the American Academy of Sleep Medicine (AASM) guidelines. Nap opportunities lasted 40 minutes. According to the guidelines, each nap opportunity should be terminated in 20 minutes if sleep is not documented. The definition of a sleep-onset REM period is the occurrence of REM sleep within 15 minutes of sleep onset. The reported average sleep-onset latency of 6.5 minutes is wrong (the correct average is 5.5 minutes). Finally the perception of sleep on the naps is not critical to the interpretation of the MSLT.

236. Answer: A

EDUCATIONAL OBJECTIVE: To appreciate sleep drug-induced alterations in sleep architecture.

EXPLANATION: Drugs agonizing the gamma amino butyric acid (GABA) and benzodiazepine (BZD) receptors potentially suppress REM sleep. However, as a group, barbiturate ingestion produces the most suppression. BZDs tend to suppress slow-wave activity to a greater extent compared to barbiturates and REM sleep to a lesser extent. The BZD receptor agonist zaleplon was not found to suppress REM sleep in clinical trials on patients with primary insomnia. Similarly, buspirone has not been shown to alter sleep architecture.

237. Answer: B

EDUCATIONAL OBJECTIVE: To understand the relationship between arterial blood gases and sleep-disordered breathing.

EXPLANATION: The patient described above is a young man with snoring and possibly mild sleep apnea. He is not obese, does not apparently have chronic obstructive lung disease, a metabolic disorder, a history of stroke, or neuromuscular disorder. There are obstructive components to his breathing disorder that essentially define the clinical problem. Negative intrathoracic pressure sometimes forces the contents of the stomach distally and causes gastroesophageal reflux and/or heartburn. In turn, gastroesophageal reflux can provoke central apnea episodes. There is no reason to expect that this patient has either high or low blood carbon dioxide (CO_2) levels.

238. Answer: D

EDUCATIONAL OBJECTIVE: To understand the relationship between chronic obstructive pulmonary disease and insomnia.

EXPLANATION: The patient described above has chronic obstructive pulmonary disease. He is not overweight and likely has emphesema rather than chronic bronchitis. The nocturnal cough is typical, especially early in the night, due to secretions. However, later in the night he most likely becomes hyperinflated due to expiratory resistance and awakens with dyspnea. The usual sleep complaint among patients afflicted with these problems is insomnia. If his insomnia were produced by major depressive disorder, we would not expect a complaint of awakening with gasping for breath. If the patient had severe undiagnosed obstructive sleep apnea, we would expect there to be snoring and/or excessive sleepiness and the bed partner would likely confirm these problems. Psychogenic choking is possible but rare and unlikely compared to this classic presentation of insomnia in a patient with lung disease.

239. Answer: A

EDUCATIONAL OBJECTIVE: To identify sleep-related changes associated with menopause.

EXPLANATION: The patient described above is postmenopausal and is not taking hormone replacement therapy. As epidemiologic data indicate, after menopause the prevalence of obstructive sleep apnea in women begins to increase and approaches the level found in men. It is likely that this patient is misattributing her blood pressure problems and that they are really related to a sleep-related breathing disorder. Daytime sleepiness associated with obstructive sleep apnea is typical in men who have been afflicted with it for many years. It is common for women, particularly if the sleep-disordered breathing is in an early stage, to manifest insomnia. Both the nocturia and increased dreaming (noticed because of REM sleep apnea–provoked awakenings) are consistent with the diagnosis. Her developing memory problems and inability to work effectively late into the night are characteristic of obstructive sleep apnea. Because she is a high-functioning individual in a demanding profession, she is more likely to notice any compromise in cognitive functions. It is possible that she has bipolar disorder; however, the history does not involve a description of mania, hypomania, dysthymia, or mood swings. Similarly, Alzheimer disease is possible but unlikely because it does not explain the insomnia, nocturia, and increased dreaming.

240. Answer: D

EDUCATIONAL OBJECTIVE: To identify causes of daytime sleepiness.

EXPLANATION: This is a young adult, healthy, married woman who suddenly is afflicted with severe sleepiness. She has good eating, sleeping, and exercise habits. There is no family history or risk factors for sleep-disordered breathing or narcolepsy. Depression screening was negative and drug abuse seems unlikely. No history of episodic bouts of sleepiness, hyperphagia, or hypersexuality is present to suggest Kleine–Levin syndrome. No recent accident, head trauma, or hypothalamic insult is noted to suggest induced idiopathic hypersomnia (possible if post viral) or idiopathic torpor (which is extremely rare). The decision to test for narcolepsy with overnight polysomnography followed by a multiple sleep latency test is sound; however, the fact that she cancelled is mostly likely due to her finding out that she is pregnant. It is common that the sleepiness precedes knowing about a pregnancy and the first trimester is associated with extreme sleepiness due to hormonal changes.

241. Answer: C

EDUCATIONAL OBJECTIVE: To elucidate the two-factor model governing sleep and wakefulness.

EXPLANATION: The homeostatic drive to sleep increases as a function of duration of wakefulness. To offset this sleep drive, the circadian (approximately day long) pacemaker of the hypothalamic suprachiasmatic nucleus (SCN) produces an alertness signal that helps maintain an even wake propensity across the day. At dusk, melatonin levels begin to rise and when they finally reach some critical level, SCN output is reduced. This in turn, allows the homeostatic drive to assert itself, the individual becomes sleepy, falls asleep, and begins to dissipate the sleep drive. Cortisol is released mainly upon awaking in the morning or when something very stressful happens, rather than being released in an increasing level across the day. Finally, the homeostatic mechanism does not episodically decrease in response to metabolic factors and any downregulation is likely to be gradual and continuous.

242. Answer: D

EDUCATIONAL OBJECTIVE: To describe the prevailing neurophysiologically derived theory of dream formation.

EXPLANATION: Neurophysiologic theory posits that REM sleep–related pontine activation ascends to the lateral geniculate and subsequently activates the occipital cortex. In animals, a neuronal discharge called ponto-geniculo-occipital (PGO) spikes occurs in bursts just before the eye movements in REM sleep. In humans, the eye movements occurring during REM sleep have been associated with changes in the direction of gaze during dreaming, that is, attempts to look at things in the dream sequence. It is believed that the neuronal activation pattern in the cortex triggers an attempt to interpret the incoming stimulation as though it were sensory. In doing so recent memories are released and the brain does its best to read meaning into the signals. Ultimately, a dream is synthesized. This theory is called the activation-synthesis hypothesis and was enunciated by Hobson and McCarley. Memories, as far as we know, are not activated by cerebellar inhibition, and the notion that dreams are archetypal racial memories is Jungian theory. There are dream theories concerning memory encoding; however, this is not the premise of the activation-synthesis hypothesis.

243. Answer: A

EDUCATIONAL OBJECTIVE: To describe the changes in sleep macro- and microarchitecture associated with depression.

EXPLANATION: Major depressive disorders are associated with many polysomnographically discernable alterations. Most of these physiologic characteristics are not specific for depression but frequently observed. They include short REM sleep latency, decreased slow-wave sleep, a shift of slow-wave sleep preponderance to the second NREM–REM cycle, difficulty initiating sleep, difficulty maintaining sleep, early morning awakening with difficulty returning to sleep, and increased electroencephalographic (EEG) beta activity during sleep.

244. Answer: C

EDUCATIONAL OBJECTIVE: To appreciate the diagnostic criteria for narcolepsy.

EXPLANATION: Clinical history suggests several sleep disorders, one of which is narcolepsy. Both hypnagogic hallucinations and sleep paralysis are part of the tetrad of ancillary symptoms associated with narcolepsy (excessive sleepiness, cataplexy, sleep paralysis, and hypnagogic or hypnapompic hallucinations). Overnight polysomnography also suggests narcolepsy; however, by itself it is not definitive. The short REM sleep latency is typical; however, it would be more convincing if the REM sleep latency was 20 minutes or less on the overnight sleep study. Sleep-related teeth grinding confirmed the presence of sleep bruxism and the complaint of nightmares may suggest some other REM sleep disturbance. However, sleep-disordered breathing levels were minimal (notwithstanding admission of snoring). To have confirmed the diagnosis of narcolepsy with multiple sleep latency testing (MSLT) would require REM sleep occurring on two of the nap opportunities. The MSLT results would not completely rule out narcolepsy even if the test had been performed properly. Minor errors included having the first test session start time at 8:15 a.m. rather than 8:00 a.m., prematurely terminating the second nap opportunity at 10:20 a.m. rather than at 10:25 a.m., and starting the third nap session at 12:28 p.m. rather than at 12:00 p.m. However, the major procedural flaw that renders this MSLT inconclusive was not conducting a fifth nap opportunity, which is required if there was only one nap with REM in the first four test sessions.

245. Answer: C

EDUCATIONAL OBJECTIVE: To identify characteristics associated with REM sleep behavior disorder (RBD) compared to other forms of out-of-bed behaviors during sleep.

EXPLANATION: The description of the sleep-related behavioral event fits with a diagnosis of RBD. Many antidepressants (selective serotonin reuptake inhibitors, tricyclic antidepressants, and monoamine oxidase inhibitors) are known to provoke RBD. The patient's comorbidity and family history do not constitute known risk factors (the way a neurodegenerative disease would), and although sleepwalking can be associated with sleeping pill ingestion, it is more common when short-acting drugs are used. The episode was clearly associated with a dream that favors RBD over sleepwalking, epilepsy, and fugue (for which the sleeper is usually amnesic). Finally, RBD is commonly associated with injury and may be prodromal for Parkinson disease, not for a recurrence of depression.

246. Answer: A

EDUCATIONAL OBJECTIVE: To distinguish between normal and abnormal electroencephalographic (EEG) patterns.

EXPLANATION: The polysomnographic sample shows a brief snapshot of mu rhythm (sometimes called wickets). Mu rhythm is composed of 7 to 11 Hz arch-shaped waves that occur in brief trains. They can be seen most clearly on recordings from central derivations during wakefulness, sleep stage N1, and sleep stage N2. They typically occur early in the night and disappear. Most importantly, they are a normal EEG variant and neither represent pathology nor require treatment.

247. Answer: A

EDUCATIONAL OBJECTIVE: To describe the ontogenetic pattern of sleep architecture.

EXPLANATION: Active sleep declines from 50% to 33% of total sleep time from birth to the end of the first year. At 10 to 12 weeks a stable diurnal distribution of sleep and wake develops. Sleep periods during this period are marked by a regular alteration of first active sleep and then quiet sleep. Periodic breathing is common at birth during active sleep but becomes rare after 7 weeks of age. There is a gradual consolidation of the multiphasic sleep pattern between ages 1 and 6 months. By age 6 months, entry to sleep via active sleep declines to approximately 18% of episodes. REM sleep remains stable at 20% to 25% of total sleep time during adulthood and slowly declines to less than 15% after age 65 years. Sleep patterns for men and women are remarkably similar throughout the lifespan with women possibly retaining their REM and N3 sleep longer.

248. Answer: A

EDUCATIONAL OBJECTIVE: To differentiate between different types of behavioral parasomnias.

EXPLANATION: REM sleep behavior disorder (RBD) is associated with posttraumatic stress disorder and the use of many antidepressants. The sleepers frequently injure themselves during the enactment of a dream. By contrast, sleepwalkers usually awaken somewhere or are awakened by someone and are confused, do not recall a dream, and do not remember how they got to the place that they find themselves. Sleepwalking can be provoked by benzodiazepine receptor agonists (BZRAs) and alcohol; however, injury is usually less likely and severe than in patients with RBD. Dopamine agonists are known to exacerbate compulsive behaviors (e.g., gambling) and sleep attacks, not dream enactments. Most association between dopamine agonists and dream enactment is confounded by comorbid Parkinson disease.

249. Answer: A

EDUCATIONAL OBJECTIVE: To identify the features of cognitive behavioral therapy for insomnia (CBT-I).

EXPLANATION: CBT-I usually begins with an assessment of the elements of the client's insomnia. Psychoeducational components include identifying sleep hygiene issues and working out a timetable for their correction, dispelling erroneous ideas about sleep and insomnia (e.g., making yourself tired by exercising before sleep will help you fall asleep), and promoting realistic expectations about the rate and course of therapeutic success. If the client has maladaptive conditioned associations with sleep onset, stimulus control therapy is employed to help associate the bed and bedroom with rapidly falling asleep. This behavioral therapy developed by Bootzin is also sometimes paired with Speilman's sleep restriction therapy, another behavioral technique designed to increase sleep efficiency. Although relaxation training is sometimes used as part of CBT-I; eye movement desensitization and reprocessing is used for posttraumatic stress disorder (PTSD); transactional analysis is used for psychotherapy, counseling, and education; and systematic desensitization is used to overcome phobia.

250. Answer: C

EDUCATIONAL OBJECTIVE: To enumerate proper electroencephalographic (EEG) sleep recording technique according to the American Academy of Sleep Medicine (AASM).

EXPLANATION: The *AASM Manual* specifies three EEG recording channels. Recommended channels include F4, C4, and O2, all referenced to the left mastoid (M1). Backup electrodes at homologous sites can be used, as needed or preferred. Alternatively, one can opt to record FZ-CZ, CZ-OZ, and C3-M1. Filtering for EEG channels should allow bandpass from 0.3 to 35 Hz. Thus, in the example above, channel 1 is inappropriate because FZ-F3 is not a recommended electrode combination and channel 2 has an incorrect low-frequency setting. Channel 3 provides a proper electrode pair combination for the alternative central to occipital midline derivation and the bandpass from 0.3 to 35 Hz is correct.

251. Answer: B

EDUCATIONAL OBJECTIVE: To understand the dynamics of shift work sleep disorder in terms of homeostatic and circadian drives.

EXPLANATION: The patient described above is a very conscientious shift worker who is trying her best to maintain a sleep–wake routine. She is not flip-flopping her sleep–wake cycle between workdays and off days; however, her sleep quality and quantity are deteriorating. Her gastrointestinal problems, musculoskeletal discomfort, and anxiety are likely sequelae of the erosion of her ability to attain adequate, good-quality sleep. During the overnight period, she has increasing homeostatic drive to sleep; however, her wakefulness propensity is not maintained evenly because a circadian alerting signal from her suprachiasmatic nucleus is likely absent. Thus, she becomes progressively sleepier as the night wears on. To maintain alertness, she judiciously self-administers the stimulant caffeine in the form of 1 to 2 cups of coffee. Soon after she returns home after work, her homeostatic drive to sleep is fully realized and even though her circadian alertness signal is becoming active, her drive to sleep wins out. However, after sleeping 3 to 4 hours, her homeostatic sleep drive is half or less than it was at bedtime and unfortunately the circadian altering signal is increasing and consequently now interfering with sleep continuity. Cortisol has not likely shifted and the homeostatic drive would shift due to food intake or bright light. While environmental factors could be playing a role, the strongest influence is likely from changes in homeostatic and circadian influences.

252. Answer: A

EDUCATIONAL OBJECTIVE: To describe what is known concerning pharmacologic nightmare induction and treatment.

EXPLANATION: It is well documented that beta-blockers can induce nightmares. Both metoprolol and propanolol ingestion are associated with provoking or exacerbating nightmare experiences. By contrast, prazosin provided relief from nightmare distress in randomized clinical trials. Although amphetamine withdrawal can provoke nightmares, antipsychotic treatment in pilot studies has used atypical, rather than traditional, neuroleptics. Anticholinergic drugs would likely suppress REM sleep and should not, as a class, provoke nightmares and one would not likely benefit from taking methylxantines stimulants. Finally, histamine antagonists, not agonists, have been tried experimentally for nightmare treatment.

253. Answer: C

EDUCATIONAL OBJECTIVE: To identify the underlying mechanisms that generate physiologic phenomena correlated with and pathophysiology associated with slow-wave sleep.

EXPLANATION: Steriades et al. have identified gamma aminobutyric acid (GABA)ergic neurons and thalamocortical relay nuclei that appear to be responsible for generating slow-wave activity that can be recorded from the cortex and surface of the scalp. Although slow-wave sleep is highly associated with the release of growth hormone, it is not controlled by the growth hormone. Suppressing slow-wave sleep reduces growth hormone release. It is true that consistently depriving slow-wave sleep is difficult and that most of the slow-wave sleep occurs early in the night. However, slow-wave activity is not responsible for circadian regulation but rather may reflect homeostatic drive for sleep. Finally, while both sleepwalking and sleep terrors usually arise from slow-wave sleep, rhythmic movement disorders (i.e., jactatio capitis nocturna) characteristically occur at the sleep–wake transition.

254. Answer: D

EDUCATIONAL OBJECTIVE: To understand some key concepts developed at the 2005 National Institutes of Health (NIH) State-of-the-Science Conference on insomnia.

EXPLANATION: The 2005 NIH State-of-the-Science Conference on insomnia produced a significant number of paradigm shifts in our conceptualization about causes and treatments of disorders of initiating and maintaining sleep. Perhaps the most fundamental was the shift away from considering insomnia as either primary or secondary to considering it primary or comorbid. The overarching feeling was that the implicit message of calling the disorder secondary insomnia was that the cause should be treated and not the insomnia. However, years of experience reveal that treating the cause (even successfully) does not necessarily relieve the insomnia. Furthermore, there is commonly a synergy between the insomnia and the comorbid condition such that deterioration of sleep can exacerbate the other condition. Therefore, using the term comorbid rather than secondary was recommended. Pharmacotherapeutic agents have now been developed and approved for long-term use, including benzodiazepine receptor agonists and synthetic melatonin agonists. The conceptualization that insomnia be treated as a symptom and that treatment be exclusively directed at the underlying cause has been completely reversed. Symptomatic treatment is now completely acceptable; the days of monotherapy have ended. Finally, behavioral treatments are highly recommended because randomized controlled trials clearly demonstrate their efficacy and safety.

255. Answer: C

EDUCATIONAL OBJECTIVE: To describe appropriate follow-up procedures for patients with obstructive sleep apnea whose job may affect public safety.

EXPLANATION: The patient described above needs to be evaluated to continue with his current job. He was diagnosed with obstructive sleep apnea and treated with continuous positive airway pressure (CPAP) therapy. His desire and agenda is to continue working; therefore, self-report for sleepiness, quality of life, therapy utilization, and overall function would be suspect. CPAP therapy can be very effective for treating sleep apnea; however, documentation of use must be objective in this case. Therefore, the patient should be using a CPAP machine that allows full disclosure of utilization statistics and these data should be downloaded and reviewed by the clinician to assure adherence to therapy. An objective test of alertness would also provide useful information. This can be obtained with a maintenance of wakefulness test (MWT) to assure that the patient can remain awake even in nonstimulating, soporific circumstances. A urine drug screen for stimulants should be collected as well. The multiple sleep latency test (MSLT) is more appropriate for diagnosing narcolepsy or showing that an individual can rapidly fall asleep. If MSLT were given to this patient, he would probably not try to fall asleep but rather try to remain awake and therefore be doing an MWT notwithstanding the clinician's instructions. The Epworth Sleepiness Scale relies on self-report and thus is of limited utility in this case. By contrast, the psychomotor vigilance test might be a good idea; however, it is not widely recognized by regulatory authorities. A physical examination and blood work is a good idea but would not provide information needed to support the "fit for duty" judgment. Finally, the situational immobilization test is designed to diagnostically assess restless legs syndrome, not evaluation sleep apnea treatment efficacy.

256. Answer: D

EDUCATIONAL OBJECTIVE: To describe ponto-geniculo-occipital (PGO) wave role in dream generation.

EXPLANATION: Hobson and McCarley's activation-synthesis hypothesis of dream formation posits that brainstem activation ascends through neuronal pathways to the lateral geniculate nuclei where it then continues and ultimately activates the occipital (visual) cortex. This excitation produces dream imagery and excites memories. The brain then makes its best attempt to generate a context to make sense out of these random activations which are interpreted as sensory input. The resultant synthesis takes its form as a dream. The activation does not release drive states, and dream elements concerning forbidden wish and desire are part of Freudian theory. Organ systems may indeed provide brain input and ultimately become part of the synthesis but this is not the crux of the theory. Finally, notions concerning unconscious representations of prototypical archetypes fall in the domain of Jungian dream theory.

257. Answer: C

EDUCATIONAL OBJECTIVE: To describe the hypothalamic dynamics associated with NREM sleep.

EXPLANATION: The ventrolateral preoptic nucleus (VLPO), referred to by Saper as the sleep switch, is thought to be involved with the regulation of sleep and circadian rhythms. This hypothalamic group of neurons decreases activity in response to noradrenaline and acetylcholine but can be activated by prostaglandin D2. Activity is most prominent during NREM sleep and appears to inhibit other neurons that are involved with the generation of wakefulness. VLPO releases galanin and gamma aminobutyric acid (GABA) and thereby inhibits the tubero-mammillary nucleus, raphe, and locus coeruleus. This circuitry is postulated as crucial for the smooth, stable, and complete changes in sleep and wakeful states that are portrayed as analogous to a flip-flop switch.

258. Answer: A

EDUCATIONAL OBJECTIVE: To enumerate the requirements of the *American Academy of Sleep Medicine (AASM) Manual* for digital polysomnographic sampling rates.

EXPLANATION: The minimum sampling rate for both electroencephalographic (EEG) and electrooculographic (EOG) signals is 200 Hz. Sampling rates for EEG are not based on technologic limitations of the equipment but rather derive from requirements needed to reconstruct the signal for visual viewing. For frequency analysis one only needs to sample at two to three times the maximum waveform frequency to be deconstructed. The minimum sampling rate for respiratory channels (airflow, nasal pressure, esophageal pressure, rib cage movement, and abdominal movement) is 25 Hz, not 1 Hz.

259. Answer: A

EDUCATIONAL OBJECTIVE: To understand the period of the circadian rhythm.

EXPLANATION: For many years it was widely believed that the period of the human circadian rhythm was close to 25 or 26 hours. This view was based in part on temperature rhythms recorded during temporal isolation studies performed in caves, bunkers, and chronobiology research institutes. In such studies, individuals were prevented from knowing the actual time and were allowed to "free run"; that is, to set their own bedtimes and arising times. However, when the constant routine paradigm was developed, circadian period estimated from the temperature cycle was found to be very close to 24 hours. In the original cave and bunker studies, disentrainment was found between the sleep–wake cycle and the temperature rhythm such that the sleep–wake cycle began accelerating its magnitude of phase delay after several days. Disentrainment and forced desynchrony do not occur unprovoked during the constant routine procedure. Finally, although temperature amplitude flattening sometimes occurs, most individuals do not phase advance their sleep–wake cycle.

260. Answer: A

EDUCATIONAL OBJECTIVE: To identify factors involved in setting and resetting the sleep–wake rhythm.

EXPLANATION: There are multiple factors that can influence the sleep–wake rhythm. These factors are called zeitgebers (time givers) and some are considered strong and others weak. Bright light appears to be the strongest factor. It can stop, phase advance, or phase delay the sleep–wake cycle. There is also some evidence that social cues may act as strong zeitgebers, especially in the absence of light variation. Exercise and eating are not considered strong influences on sleep–wake circadian rhythmicity.

261. Answer: D

EDUCATIONAL OBJECTIVE: To understand dynamics of seasonal affective disorder.

EXPLANATION: Although Laguna, California, is definitely groovy, people still get depressed. Also, while her diet and lifestyle may have improved, and there is no question that winters are not as cold in Southern California than in Oslo, her improved mood more likely results from decreased seasonal affective disorder. The difference in day length between winter and summer is much more extreme in Norway and the circadian component of seasonal affective disorder plays a more pronounced role.

262. Answer: C

EDUCATIONAL OBJECTIVE: To identify sleep-coupled endocrine release, in particular, growth hormone's coupling with slow-wave sleep.

EXPLANATION: Growth hormone release is coupled with stage N3 sleep; therefore, most of its release occurs early in the night. It is not tied to circadian variation and thus would not likely be uncoupled by rapid travel through time zones (i.e., jet lag).

263. Answer: C

EDUCATIONAL OBJECTIVE: To describe the circadian timing of cortisol release.

EXPLANATION: Under normal circumstances, cortisol peaks in the morning approximately at the time of awakening. Cortisol will also increase in response to stress and is sometimes referred to as the stress hormone. For this reason, it is sometimes jokingly explained that the coincidence between peak hormone release and the end of the sleep period is because getting out of bed in the morning is the most stressful thing one does all day.

264. Answer: D

EDUCATIONAL OBJECTIVE: To identify the cyclic alternating pattern (CAP) and understand its relationship to sleep instability.

EXPLANATION: Normal sleep macroarchitecture in a patient complaining of insomnia is the basis of diagnosing paradoxical insomnia. Previously this condition was termed insomnia without objective complaint or even more derisively as pseudoinsomnia. However, the more sensitive microarchitectural electroencephalographic (EEG) features can sometimes be correlated with reported difficulty initiating and/or maintaining sleep. Such features include alpha-delta sleep, microarousals, and CAP. The example provided here depicts CAP. By contrast, the mu rhythm (sometimes called wickets because of its archiform shape similar to croquet wickets) is a 7- to 11-cycle normal variant of sleep that is not correlated clinically with insomnia complaints. Periorbital integrated potentials are brief bursts recordable just before rapid eye movements from electrodes placed near the eye that were once thought to possibly represent a human equivalent to ponto-geniculo-occipital (PGO) spikes.

265. Answer: D

EDUCATIONAL OBJECTIVE: To identify probable parasomnias and recognize their polysomnographic correlates.

EXPLANATION: The tracing shown in this example illustrates teeth grinding (sleep bruxism). Under normal circumstances, the etiology of sleep bruxism is not known; however, stress is a strongly suspected contributing factor. Nonetheless, parasomnias often occur as a result of drug abuse. Amphetamine, cocaine, ecstasy, and other stimulant use can be associated with gnawing, teeth clenching, teeth grinding, rhythmic movement disorder, and sleep-related dissociative behaviors.

266. Answer: A

EDUCATIONAL OBJECTIVE: To identify and differentiate sweat artifact from other polysomnographic phenomena.

EXPLANATION: The patient described here has chronic obstructive pulmonary disease and although he does not have problems with increased inspiratory resistance, he does have increased expiratory resistance. As he becomes hyperinflated late in the night, respiratory effort provokes nocturnal sweating and the polysomnographic tracing shows what is sometimes mistakenly scored as slow-wave activity. The tight coupling with airflow provides evidence that it is not delta activity (additionally the frequency is too low and the waveform is too rhythmic) or periodic lateralizing epileptiform discharges (PLEDs) (he does not have severe brain damage and/or is not in coma). Finally, hypothyroidism (not hyperthyroidism) might increase stage N3 sleep but these are not delta waves.

267. Answer: B

EDUCATIONAL OBJECTIVE: To understand nocturnal seizure previously labeled nocturnal paroxysmal dystonia and recognize subtle electroencephalographic (EEG) abnormalities.

EXPLANATION: The polysomnographic sample shows several phantom spikes occurring in isolation and embedded within higher-amplitude waveforms. For many years, nocturnal paroxysmal dystonia was suspected to arise from subcortical or frontal lobe seizures; however, data were lacking because scalp recordings are often not sensitive enough to reveal such pathophysiologies. In the case described above and depicted in the sample, very subtle EEG anomalies can be seen on close inspection (note bottom channel at far left, bottom channel approximately midway through trace, and embedded in theta wave burst on all channels at the right). The sample shows neither flattening in temporal lobe EEG nor clear sharp waves. Finally, sawtooth theta is an REM, not NREM, waveform.

268. Answer: B

EDUCATIONAL OBJECTIVE: To recognize drug-induced electroencephalographic (EEG) abnormalities.

EXPLANATION: The sample polysomnographic tracing illustrates excessive sleep spindle activity. The spindles are both too frequent and high amplitude. The most common cause for this is chronic and/or high-dose ingestion of drugs activating the gamma aminobutyric acid (GABA)-A receptor complex, most notably, benzodiazepines. Without tracings of respiratory activity it is not clear whether or not sleep-disordered breathing is present. Finally, the sample does not depict REM sleep; therefore, it is not possible to determine from this sample if muscle augmentation during REM sleep is present.

269. Answer: A

EDUCATIONAL OBJECTIVE: To recognize drug-induced electroencephalographic (EEG) abnormalities.

EXPLANATION: Selective serotonin reuptake inhibitors like fluoxetine and tricyclic antidepressants like clomipramine may increase electromyographic (EMG) bursts, eye movement activity in NREM, and fast EEG activity. We see here an example of eye movement activity intruding into NREM sleep. While it is possible that this was produced by clomipramine, it is more likely a result of fluoxetine ingestion. In fact, this type of activity is so commonly produced by fluoxetine that it is referred to as Prozac eyes by some clinicians. If the patient had been taking benzodiazepines, we would expect to see increased sleep spindle activity. Finally, there is no such thing as a beta encephalon agonist.

270. Answer: C

EDUCATIONAL OBJECTIVE: To recognize electroencephalographic (EEG) correlates of wakefulness and sleep.

EXPLANATION: The polysomnographic sample depicts a classic example of sleep onset. Note the prominent alpha EEG activity giving way to lower-voltage, mixed-frequency activity. Concurrently, slow rolling eye movements emerge and chin electromyographic (EMG) tone diminishes. Although this epoch would be scored overall as wakefulness because alpha EEG comprises more than 50% of the sample, the fact that the transition to sleep is occurring makes that a better answer. This sample shows very distinct EEG waveforms, not an ambiguous pattern typical in patients with severe sleep apnea. Finally, copious alpha EEG activity is present, the eye movements are slow rather than rapid, and chin EMG tone is high; consequently, this is not an example of REM sleep.

271. Answer: A

EDUCATIONAL OBJECTIVE: To recognize sleep-related respiratory events.

EXPLANATION: The polysomnographic sample depicted in this illustration, according to the *American Academy of Sleep Medicine (AASM) Scoring Manual,* would be classified as a respiratory effort–related arousal or as a hypopnea (using the alternate definition). We see a reduction in airflow, presumably due to increased airway resistance, notwithstanding continued respiratory effort (note diaphragmatic movement continues without interruption). Finally, a burst of chin electromyographic (EMG) activity occurs and normal-amplitude airflow signals resume. The presumption here is that an arousal occurred. The close temporal coincidence between the chin EMG burst and the termination of flow limitation argues against the event being spontaneous. Because there is little or no oxygen desaturation (certainly less than 4%) associated with this sleep-related respiratory event, it does not meet the Centers for Medicare and Medicaid Services (CMS) criteria for classification as a hypopnea. Finally, if this event was a result of reduced respiratory set point, we would expect to see a central-type sleep-disordered breathing event in which there would be a reduction or cessation of both airflow and effort.

272. Answer: D

EDUCATIONAL OBJECTIVE: To identify sleep stages and appreciate their contribution to overall normal sleep composition.

EXPLANATION: The polysomnographic activity shown here illustrates the classic stage N2 pattern. Note the sleep spindle in the first third of the epoch and K-complex during the final fifth of the sample. Chin electromyographic (EMG) tone is high and no eye movements are noted. In a healthy young adult, stage N2 sleep comprises 45% to 55% of the night's sleep.

273. Answer: D

EDUCATIONAL OBJECTIVE: To appreciate sleep stage patterns and acute polysomnographic events.

EXPLANATION: The polysomnographic sample depicted here would be scored as REM sleep; however, during the final moments shown in this tracing (at the far right), a central nervous system arousal occurs, recognizable by the sudden burst in alpha electroencephalographic (EEG) activity and a slight increase in chin electromyographic (EMG) tone.

274. Answer: C

EDUCATIONAL OBJECTIVE: To recognize sleep stage characteristics.

EXPLANATION: The sample tracing shows sleep stage N1 activity. We see a low-voltage, mixed-frequency background, some chin electromyographic (EMG) tone, and possible slow eye movements. The absence of rapid eye movements, sleep spindles, K-complexes, and slow-wave activity rules out stages R, N2, and N3 sleep.

275. Answer: B

EDUCATIONAL OBJECTIVE: To recognize sleep stage characteristics.

EXPLANATION: The sample tracing shows sleep stage N3 activity. We see a continual high-voltage, low-frequency slow-wave activity on both electroencephalographic (EEG) and electrooculographic (EOG) channels. Activity on EOG channels is in phase and therefore represents frontal slow waves being sensed by electrodes on the outer canthi of left and right eyes. This particular example of stage N3 would previously have been classified as stage 4 sleep using the Rechtschaffen and Kales system. It is not classified as N4 because no such classification exists in either the new or old scoring systems.

276. Answer: C

EDUCATIONAL OBJECTIVE: To recognize polysomnographic events.

EXPLANATION: The sample illustrates a leg movement occurring just before a central nervous system arousal. Although the background sleep stage is NREM, the main feature of this illustration is the sleep continuity disturbance associated with the electromyographic (EMG) burst recorded from the anterior tibialis.

277. Answer: A

EDUCATIONAL OBJECTIVE: To recognize polysomnographic events.

EXPLANATION: This sample shows a classic example of an episode of obstructive sleep apnea. Note the complete cessation of airflow notwithstanding continued respiratory effort indicated by diaphragmatic motion. The tracing shows paradoxical (asynchronous) movement of the rib cage and abdomen that further attests to there being an airway obstruction as the cause of airflow cessation. The unusual tracing on the electrocardiographic (ECG) channel is artifact produced by movement.